The First Year of Nursing

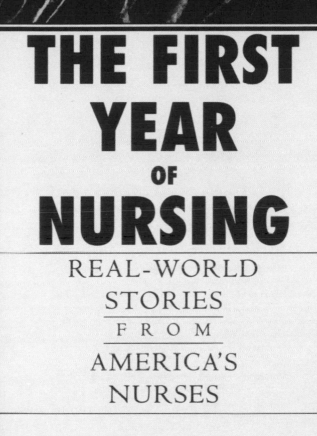

THE FIRST
YEAR
OF
NURSING

REAL-WORLD

STORIES

FROM

AMERICA'S

NURSES

Edited by

BARBARA FINKELSTEIN

WALKER AND COMPANY
NEW YORK

Copyright © 1996 by Walker and Company

Many of the names used in the book are fictitious.

First published in the United States of America in 1996 by
Walker Publishing Company, Inc.

Published simultaneously in Canada by Thomas Allen & Son Canada,
Limited, Markham, Ontario

Library of Congress Cataloging-in-Publication Data
The first year of nursing: real-world stories from America's nurses/
edited by Barbara Finkelstein.
        p.   cm.
Includes bibliographical references and index.
ISBN 0-8027-1296-7 (hardcover). —ISBN 0-8027-7428-8 (pbk.)
    1. Nursing—Anecdotes.   I. Finkelstein, Barbara, 1937–
                    RT61.F47   1996
        610.73—dc20   96-12903   CIP

Printed in the United States of America

2   4   6   8   10   9   7   5   3   1

Dedicated to Max

Contents

viii   *Contents*

Foreword

ANNE GRISWOLD PEIRCE, R.N., PH.D.

Almost everyone knows at least one nurse, but few people outside the profession know what nurses actually do. Most of the public's concepts of nursing come from novels or from TV shows like *E.R.* and *Chicago Hope*. Despite the changes that have taken place in the health-care industry, many people still have a stereotyped view of nurses: as women in white uniforms who work in hospitals at simple tasks like changing bedpans and giving sponge baths. But nurses can be male or female; they work in many settings besides hospitals; and even though nursing is, to some degree, a task-oriented profession, it also demands diagnostic expertise, technical skill, and psychological insight.

Nursing came of age in 1854 in the Crimea when Florence Nightingale brought hygienic nursing techniques to the battlefield. Before her appearance on the health-care scene, the nurse was, in the words of social biographer Lytton Strachey, "a coarse old woman, always ignorant, usually dirty, often brutal, a Mrs. Gamp, in bunched-up sordid garments, tippling at the brandy bottle or indulging in worse irregularities." Nightingale was the first person to argue in favor of consistent, scientific care. Indeed, her most persuasive arguments were grounded in statistics: She reported that mortality declined *1,000 percent* after she installed trained nurses in the hospitals at Scutari, Turkey. Florence Nightingale's revolutionary work ultimately won her membership in England's Royal Academy of Statisticians—the only woman in the group.

From the hospital, nurses branched out into communities, forming visiting nurse associations and other nonhospital-based nursing organizations. Today nurses work in schools, clinics, major corporations, mobile vans, community centers, and, as you will read in *The First Year of Nursing,* everywhere from a nursing home in New Jersey to a Cambodian refugee camp on the Thai border.

Nurses do everything. In the hospital, they start and maintain intra-venous lines (IVs). They defibrillate (stop the uncontrolled twitching of the heart muscle using electroshock) and resuscitate people in cardiac arrest. These and the many other tasks nurses perform require knowledge and intelligence. Any nurse will tell you that even the contents of a bedpan can be important; the nurse's observant eye can spot a change in urine or bowel habits that may signal serious complications of disease and surgery.

Inside and outside the hospital, nurse-midwives deliver babies and provide pre- and postnatal care to mothers. Nurse anesthetists give the majority of surgical anesthesia in the United States. Nurse practitioners provide primary care to growing numbers of health-care consumers. School nurses screen children for physical and emotional illnesses. Hospice nurses provide care and comfort to the dying. And through home visits, visiting nurses make it possi-ble for people to receive care in their own home.

While the knowledge required to become a nurse takes several years of education, the application of that schooling is an art acquired only with experience. The first year of nursing is really a postgraduate course in the art of nursing. Consider, for example, the hospitalized man who complains that he is cold. Common sense might tell us that the room is cold and the patient needs another blanket. A textbook diagnosis may suggest that the patient's complaint indicates fever. Only a sensitive, experienced nurse, however, will be able to discern when the patient's complaint is a sign that he is scared and lonely, in need of the warmth of human contact.

In her or his first year, the nurse hones the fundamental skills needed for a career in nursing. During this time, the new nurse gains confidence and eventually, a love of the profession. The first year also reminds nurses that an effective nurse keeps learning. Nursing cannot be mastered in four, eight, or sixteen years. It is a lifelong education.

Nurses have the rare privilege of interacting with a succession of people in an intimate relationship, one full of humor, sadness, life, and death. It is a relationship that many people outside the profession can only begin to imagine, but that nurses come to know heart, mind, body, and soul.

Anne Griswold Peirce, R.N., Ph.D., is Director of Doctoral Studies at Columbia University's School of Nursing in New York City.

Acknowledgments

Grateful acknowledgment to the following people for helping me find some of the nurses interviewed here: Dr. Neil Halpern, Marcie Horowitz, Eric Levy, Jean Murray, R.N., Daphna Pollack, and Mary Reynolds Powell, R.N. My thanks also to Carolyn Zagury, R.N. for suggesting a bibliography and to Pesha Rubinstein for her help in preparing this manuscript.

Introduction

As the voices in this book attest, nursing is a diverse profession. In the course of a thirty-year career, a nurse may dress battlefield wounds, medicate cancer patients, bring babies into the world, provide anesthesia during surgery, conduct psychiatric therapy, educate diabetics, detect evidence of child abuse, or lend a sympathetic ear to a young prison inmate. She—and increasingly he—may work in a variety of settings, including hospitals, the military, nursing homes, clinics, geriatric daycare centers, missionary outposts, research facilities, schools, and patients' homes.

Nursing, like medicine, has been the beneficiary of numerous social and scientific changes. Nearly thirty years ago, for example, when Leah Harrison, a child protection advocate, became a staff nurse at New York's Montefiore Medical Center, she witnessed the death of children from Wilms' tumor; today specific chemotherapeutic drugs can cure this otherwise lethal form of cancer. As little as a decade ago, mastectomy was the only viable option for women with breast cancer; today early detection through mammography, and treatment with specifically targeted, high-dose radiation, gives many more women the chance of surviving breast cancer physically intact. And, while a generation ago, diseases like diabetes and high blood pressure were a death sentence for people in their seventies and eighties, today geriatric care—more and more the province of nursing care—has helped enhance the quality of life for millions of patients.

From the nurse's point of view, nursing has evolved from an elitist profession staffed by upper- and middle-class women to a life's work performed by men and women of virtually every nationality, race, and religion. An R.N. license is frequently the ticket to a socially important, well-paid career.

The biggest change in nursing—and the one whose long-range effects are still unknown—is the delivery of health care by managed-care organizations. Managed care, which appears to be the wave of the health-care future, is, as of this writing, a controversial experiment in social reengineering. To its defenders, managed care is the best way for our society to cut extravagant health-care costs, eliminate unnecessary medical tests, and promote a "wellness" plan of good dietary habits and exercise. To its detractors, it is a business, dominated by the health insurance industry, that rations health care, takes health-care decisions out of the hands of doctors and nurses, and operates on a crass bottom-line principle. While few of the chapters here make mention of managed care—it did not exist when these nurses were rookies—it will certainly have a dramatic effect on the profession in the future. Indeed, several nurses I interviewed were distraught over the current trend by managed care outfits and budget-strapped hospitals to hire Licensed Practical Nurses (L.P.N.s) and aides instead of R.N.s.

The focus of this book, however, is not the current state of nursing, but rather the insight that nurses gained early on in the profession. Some of the experiences described here involve professional hazards or personal danger: In "A Visiting Nurse Confronts the Down and Out," Phyllis Newton had a close call while making her rounds in an area where there had been series of rapes. Barbara Hesselman Kautz recounts the ethical dilemma posed by triaging critically wounded soldiers in "The Twenty-fourth Evac: An Army Nurse's Vietnam Tour of Duty." And perhaps nobody showed more courage than Nancy Jean Murray, who, in "Desert Storm: All for One and One for All," describes how she persevered in her effort to become an army nurse despite staggering legal obstacles. The first year may have been difficult, even demoralizing, but it also strengthened these nurses in their resolve to be nurses.

Several R.N.s talk about the feelings of insecurity that come with the territory of any first job. In "Two Valuable Mistakes," Rachel Rivera talks about two unfortunate oversights she made early in her career, and about her determination not to repeat them. Ruth Adelman ("Daughters of Miriam: One Nurse's Second Home") and Dorothy Stagno ("Finding a Niche in Nursing") discuss having felt so overwhelmed by the demands of hospital nursing that they resigned their positions in order to look for other more satisfying nursing work. As Patty Tentler in "Sixth Sense: Learning to Trust Your Intuition" observes, "One of the hardest things to learn as a new nurse is what to take seriously."

In gathering interview candidates for *The First Year of Nursing*, I wanted to offer readers a representative cross-section of the nursing profession. Thus, this volume includes first-year accounts by several hospital staff nurses, a psychiatric nurse, a nurse-midwife, a visiting nurse, a nursing home nurse, two military nurses, two missionary nurses, and a nurse-practitioner. Their stories convey the humanity and wit that I have come to see are the mark and trade of a successful "nursing personality." As a writer who has

written about nurses since the 1980s, I am humbled by the forti-
tude that education and human kindness have instilled in these
eighteen women and one man, and in the many other nurses who
took the time to tell me their stories for this book. I am grateful
to all of them for working with me to turn their private memories
into personal histories.

For the sake of confidentiality, I have fictionalized the names
of all patients, doctors, and nurse colleagues mentioned herein.
Public personalities—Richard Nixon and Robert McNamara, for
example—have withstood greater scrutiny than their treatment in
this book, so I have left their names, and the names of other
historical and literary figures, unchanged. All the hospitals are real,
except where identified as fictitious. One nurse—"Naomi Shuster"—requested anonymity; all other nurses consented to the use
of real bylines.

Despite the inevitable changes in our health-care system, people
will always need nurses. A new nurse today may not get a first-
pick job in a first-pick location, but with good training and a
willingness to go where needed, she or he can offer education,
comfort, and holistic care to patients in medical centers, refugee
camps, and battle zones, in urban American neighborhoods or
farflung rural villages. To the veteran nurses in *The First Year of
Nursing*, nursing is a calling. It is the source of meaningful work,
a steady income, and a satisfying way of experiencing the wider
world.

The First Year of Nursing

1

A Glass of Milk in the Night

 GLORIA RAMSEY

The summer before I graduated from the Charles E. Gregory School of Nursing, I worked as a nurse's aide at the Hebrew Home for the Aged in Jersey City, New Jersey. I liked the place, and the place liked me. One of the administrators invited me to come back after I graduated, and I did. But after eating, drinking, and sleeping nursing for three years straight, I wanted the summer for myself. I asked to work the night shift so I could play tennis during the day. I could not think of a more perfect schedule.

I've been told that the nursing home is the lowest order of nursing. Basically, your job is to dispense medications, but you also monitor bowel movements, hang IVs, and give baths. My complaint was never with the tasks at hand, and it was certainly never with the patients.

Two patients have stayed in my mind ever since I took care of them in 1971. One was a one-hundred-year-old woman who had grown up in Jersey City precisely where the Hebrew Home now stood. The property, an area called Greenville, had been farmland back in the 1870s when she was a child. She talked about her parents' cows and how they would milk them. She had a great craving for milk and used to ask me to get her some from the kitchen. But it was against the rules to give patients food or drink after scheduled meal times. I thought that was unfair. After all, the patient *was* one hundred years old, and I felt she should be able to eat or drink whatever she wanted at this point in her life. The old woman was grateful for the milk I scavenged from the refrigerator, but she teasingly reminded me that it was not as good as the fresh milk from her parents' cows.

I witnessed a similar scenario with a 103-year-old man. He too was always hungry, and the staff would not let him have extra food either. I used to rummage through the pantry to get him a little bread and milk.

While I felt close to patients like these two very old people, I had a strained relationship with my supervisor. Miss Sprague was a black woman from the Caribbean. I am an African-American woman from the northeastern United States. We should have been natural allies because, no matter what year it is, it's a tough job market for women of color. Miss Sprague had been at the nursing home for several years when I arrived. She had a Ph.D. but hadn't been able to find work where she could put it to better use. Here I come along, a young R.N. from a pampered three-year nursing program, and I'm a threat.

From the start, I felt Miss Sprague tried to undermine me in my work. Except for having worked at the Hebrew Home as an aide, and having had the benefit of an excellent education (a non-bachelor's degree nursing program), I had no idea what was expected of me. It was Miss Sprague's job to show me the ropes. She was supposed to be my mentor. Instead, she would speak to me in a high, intimidating voice. "Any problem?" she would ask. Her tone implied that I should keep my mouth shut. I was damned if I did, damned if I didn't. Miss Sprague reported to her boss that "Miss Ramsey is not cooperative." This woman wanted me to fail, and my annual evaluation reflected her bias.

After less than a year as a staff nurse, I was offered a promotion to supervisor of the intensive care unit. In some other situation, a promotion would have been cause to celebrate. However, I simply was not prepared to take on such a big responsibility. I was in a quandary. My goal all along was to work in an ICU in New York City. The Hebrew Home had just opened its ICU, and I wanted to get some experience working there. Should I accept the promotion and get the prestige that went along with it, or should I move on to New York?

I had to talk to someone. I called the Charles E. Gregory School of Nursing and talked to the director, whom I liked and respected. She told me something I have always remembered: "Gloria, institutions use you for their own needs. You have to think about what *you* need." When she said that, I knew that taking the supervisory position would be a mistake. I didn't have the skills for it. I wouldn't have the collegial support I needed. Worst of all, I felt I would be a puppet, manipulated by a nursing administration that did not give me—a new member of the profession—the support I needed.

Before the year was out, I got a new job, this time at the Jersey City Medical Center. I stayed on the night shift so I could continue playing tennis during the day.

At Jersey City's ICU, I saw the worst of humanity. Drug addicts. Prostitutes. Gunshot victims. Here I was, a liberal, bleeding-heart black woman who had good parents, a wonderful education, and a crusading conviction to take care of the world. These patients that the ambulances carted in during the middle of the night were not lovable. The drug addicts would wake up fighting, kicking, cursing, spitting, urinating all over themselves. And if the patients were difficult, the doctors weren't always much better. One night a surgeon wheeled in a guy with a gunshot wound. He stood in the open door of the ICU, pushed the stretcher through, and said, "Take care of him!" Then he bolted.

"Holy mackerel!" I said. "What am I supposed to do?" Even though there were five other nurses with me to attach plasma and antibiotic bags to IV poles, we could not work fast enough to save the guy. He died.

After that, I thought, "There's got to be a better place to work." I wanted more for myself professionally. I wanted colleagues who practiced ethically and systems that provided me with the equipment and support I needed to do my job.

Ultimately, continuing my education saved me. From my monthly reading of the *American Journal of Nursing*, I understood that nursing was going to become more competitive, and that if I was to improve my professional standing, I had to keep acquiring new skills and advanced degrees. Moreover, I have always had a knack for removing myself from bad situations. Having a tenacious sort of personality, I believed that my job dissatisfaction lay in my environment, not in me, and not in nursing. Before the end of my second year, I decided that playing tennis by day and working as a nurse by night was getting me nowhere fast. I found a job in the NYU Medical Center ICU on the day shift, with some night-time rotation. After a year, I entered the Jersey City State College nursing program to get my baccalaureate degree. Because this institution's accreditation was pending, I decided to transfer to NYU's five-year program. The NYU program was accredited and rated number one in the country.

A lot of people thought I was crazy to bother with a five-year baccalaureate program after I had been in a diploma program for three years. They believed I was wasting my time. I told them,

"You know what, guys? I'm not in any rush. I don't want to miss a thing. So here I go again."

I can still remember walking around the NYU campus in Greenwich Village and thinking, "This is the place for me." I loved the academic atmosphere. The professors were bright and helpful, and they became my role models. Three years had passed since I first entered the profession. Finally, I had found my niche.

Despite my love for the NYU Medical Center, I wasn't always happy with the priorities there. The emphasis was on research and teaching, both of which I admired. But as a nurse, I believed we should also remember to be considerate of patients, and indeed it was the nurse's job to close curtains, shut doors, turn off lights, and let the patients sleep for a while before waking them up for their medication. I vowed to embrace the best of what I had learned at Charles E. Gregory and NYU.

People who know me well always say, "Gloria, you never give up." They're right. I always take the difficult way. If it's easy, I'm not interested. That's been true for me in matters regarding romance, money, friends, shopping, and nursing. I take the path of greatest resistance.

As an African-American woman in the health-care industry, I have no other choice. Regrettably, I face racism from every corner—from white colleagues and even from my own people.

Racism from white people is obvious. In nursing school, I remember sitting with a group of students and watching a TV program in which a black man was shining a white man's shoes. This was the late 1960s, the so-called era of black power, and I was appalled. I blurted out, "Would you just look at that!" It was clear that I thought his characterization insulting to African-American people.

One of the white students, a well-to-do young woman whose family owned horses and had servants, snapped, "Well, at least he has a job!"

I couldn't take that sitting down. "That's just fine," I said, "but society ought to offer this man more opportunities!" I said that the only reason this man was shining shoes was because he had no other choices.

This garden-variety racism is always tough to swallow, and it always puts me in a bad mood. Just imagine hailing a cab and getting passed by because you're black, then having to go to work where you have to take care of people of *all* colors.

Racism from your own people is even more pathetic.

More than twenty years ago, on one of my first days at NYU, I drove up to the parking garage in my car. I handed the black parking attendant a five-dollar bill because I did not know how much the parking spot cost. "I don't have change for this!" he yelled, waving my money around. "What do you expect *me* to do with this!" He carried on as if I had just handed him a wet sock. I said to myself, "This is the beginning of the rest of my life. This man wants me to leave. *But I'm not going.*"

I said, "Thank you very much," and I pulled my car into the first parking spot I saw. I walked away without getting change.

Twenty-two years later, I have an apartment in the Village and I'm still working at the NYU Medical Center, where the black nurses give me the same hard time that Miss Sprague gave me in 1971. When my mother died last year, one of the black clerks, a Caribbean woman, came up to me and said, "So, Glo. Are you going to sell me your car? Now that you have an inheritance, you'll be buying yourself a Lexus." Here I was in pain, crying at the drop of a hat because my mother, my best friend, was no longer physically present on this earth, and all this woman could talk about was "upscaling" myself.

Sometimes I think back to those lovely old people I knew in the Hebrew Home for the Aged. They had come a long way in their lives, and they only wanted some simple pleasures to take them to the end of their days: They wanted somebody to talk to . . . an occasional glass of milk in the night. Every so often, I ask myself what I want. I too want a few trusted souls to talk to. I want the peace of mind that comes from doing a job well and being respected for it. That's my glass of milk in the night.

Gloria Ramsey is a cooperative care nurse at New York University Hospital in New York City. As a cooperative care nurse she teaches patients' families how to care for the patient at home.

2

Two Valuable Mistakes

 RACHEL RIVERA

After my friend Diego died of AIDS, I made critical care my cause. As a nursing student at Columbia-Presbyterian in New York, I did a clinical round on the fifth floor of the Harkness Pavilion, which is the AIDS ward. I learned about infections like cytomegalovirus that affect the retina, spread to the gastrointestinal tract, and severely damage the kidneys. I studied medical interactions and the opportunistic infections that wreak havoc on the body's immune system. From my work with AIDS patients, I developed a philosophy of nursing: Quality of life is paramount. When you die is not the question; it's how you live your life that matters.

After nursing school, I moved to New Orleans to be near David and Jordan, two friends who are HIV-positive. I lived with them while I looked for a job. The South is strapped for nurses, so I had no trouble landing a position as a staff nurse at Tulane University Medical Center. I worked on a med-surg floor with overflow from other units, so we took care of everybody from cancer patients to new mothers and diabetics. Columbia's sixteen-month nursing program had given me a solid foundation in science, but I was in for a surprise when I started working in the real world.

Procedures like inserting feeding tubes I had done only once or twice before. The same was true for changing dressings, cleaning a colostomy (a bag worn after a surgical procedure that enables the contents of the lower intestine to be collected outside the body), and measuring intake and output of suction tubes. Some of these tasks were repulsive, but more shocking was the sense of overwhelming responsibility I carried with me all the time. I kept thinking, "Here I am on my own, and I have to keep this person *alive."*

A typical day meant taking care of six patients, one or two of them AIDS cases and the rest older patients with diabetes and vascular illnesses. AIDS cases in particular require a lot of antibiotics, IV fluids, and for patients who cannot ingest food by mouth, parenteral nutrition (nutrients taken into the body by means other than the digestive canal). I also hung bags of blood used in transfusions, sometimes three bags a day. This was one of the most tedious—and most psychologically demanding—jobs I had. When you hang blood, you cannot leave the room for an hour. You have to take vital signs every fifteen or thirty minutes, and once the blood is flowing, you have to watch for fever and chills, which are signs of a negative reaction to the transfusion.

The first person I hung blood for was an AIDS patient. He was so disoriented and combative that he challenged my commitment to treat each patient with dignity. He was under a Do-Not-Resuscitate order, which means the medical and nursing staff are not to take any extraordinary measures (respirator, feeding tube, or other life-support systems) to keep a patient alive.

One day he went into distress, so I called my first code. If a patient is in a crisis, you call the hospital operator, who then announces the code over a public address system. A red code means the patient is having a heart attack. A blue code means the patient is not breathing. The code team rushes in and goes to work. That was also the first time I performed CPR on a real patient. Calling a code scares me to death. I may be a wreck inside, but I'm capable and levelheaded on the outside!

I try to empathize with patients. I know it's not fun being sick. A nurse wakes you up in the middle of the night to take your vital signs. A doctor does a little poking and prodding and frequently leaves without saying a word to you.

Some patients get angry, and they take it out on the nurse. Occasionally, I have had to be stern. One of my patients was under medical orders to lie in bed with her leg elevated. She had a blood clot in her calf, and moving about could dislodge it. One morning I came in from the nursing station and found that she had gotten up and walked to the bathroom.

I thought it was time for a heart-to-heart talk. I told the patient, "If that clot dislodges, it can travel to your brain or heart and get stuck there. *You could die.* I strongly recommend that you stay in bed with your leg up, as your doctor ordered." She finally got the message and apologized. I realized that she, like many patients, did not comprehend how close to death her noncompliance had brought her.

In addition to caring for patients, nurses have to be mindful of administrative rules. For example, toward the middle of my six-month tenure at Tulane, I had a patient on a PCA, a pain-control analgesia machine that allows the patient to manage his or her own pain by pushing a button and releasing a premeasured dose of morphine. The patient is never in danger of overdosing because the PCA has a built-in regulatory safeguard. One day the doctor discontinued its use, so I separated the vial from the syringe and stuck the half-full container of morphine in my pocket. I meant to drop it off at the nurse's station, but I forgot. I was already on the bus going home when I reached for my house keys and pulled out the vial.

Like all hospitals, Tulane has a disposal protocol for narcotics. As a new staff nurse, though, I wasn't familiar with the policy. When I got home, I called the hospital and asked to speak to Melissa Cord, the charge nurse. The secretary said Melissa was writing up her reports and couldn't take my call. I explained that I had taken this PCA vial home accidentally. I noted how much morphine was still in it and said I would bring it back in the morning. The secretary promised to relay my message to Melissa.

A PCA syringe has no needle. It has a plastic screw attachment that connects to IV tubing, so I wasn't in danger of pricking myself or anybody else with it.

That afternoon, my friend Jordan had called to say that he'd had a rough day at the AIDS clinic. He had asked if I'd meet him for dinner so he could let off some steam. (I no longer stayed with Jordan and David. Now that I was working, I had my own place.) I met him at a café near my apartment, and we talked for a couple of hours.

Soon after I got home, Jordan called me to say Tulane had left *seven* messages on his answering machine. The messages were urgent, and I was to call the hospital immediately. I did.

It was eleven o'clock. Melissa, the charge nurse, insisted that I bring the vial back at once. I didn't argue. I got off the phone and called Jordan and David to see if they could drive me to the hospital. (I was not about to take the bus to Tulane late at night because I did not want to get mugged in the line of duty.)

I went up to med-surg. A platoon of hospital staff was waiting to meet me. The nursing administrator of the hospital was there. So were a security guard, the charge nurse, and all the night nurses.

I arrived at the nurses' station, put the vial down on the counter, and said, "Here it is."

Carol Burns, the nursing administrator, said, "Why didn't you return our calls?"

I told her that she had called Jordan and David's place, where I had lived before I got my own apartment. The office had my new number. In any case, I said, I was out with friends and didn't get back until late.

Ms. Burns said, "The rule is that you bring back any medication taken from the hospital immediately."

I apologized. I said I didn't know the rule.

The interrogation continued: "We were worried because you didn't bring back the morphine and you didn't return our calls."

I got offended. This was ridiculous. My colleagues had implied that I had been up to something with the morphine. What was I going to do? Pipette a couple drops into my shrimp scampi?

Melissa and Ms. Burns told me that in the future, I should bring any medication back at once. By the time they finished reprimanding me, it was one in the morning. I had to be back at work in six hours.

After all was said and done, I did not take this incident personally. Melissa had only one year's experience as a nurse, not much more than I had. Her inexperience may have caused her to handle the crisis badly. Anyway, I worked days and she worked nights, so I did not have much contact with her.

After six months in New Orleans, I decided to move to San Francisco to be with my significant other. I was leaving a job I loved, despite my falling-out with the charge nurse. In those six months, Tulane had turned me into a nurse. By the time I left, I was instructing nursing students. I had the respect of my peers. And I had learned to thread an IV into a vein. That was my proudest moment! I got so proficient that I later joined an IV team in San Francisco.

Getting a job in the Bay Area was difficult. I sent applications to twenty-two hospitals and nursing homes from San Jose to Northern California. No one called. I got a lot of nice little postcards that said, "We received your application. We will contact you immediately if your qualifications . . ." I reluctantly considered some per diem jobs. Those positions are lucrative, but they do not offer benefits or job security. I wanted both.

After a few weeks, I got a call from the Visiting Nurse Association for a case manager/R.N. position. I would have to travel to people's homes and work forty hours a week in addition to one weekend a month. The salary was bottom-of-the-barrel, as they put it, but it paid five dollars an hour more than Tulane. The VNA preferred a nurse with a full year of experience, but I think my fluency in Spanish ultimately won me the job.

I manage twenty-four patients and see a variety of illnesses. I handle all the paperwork, deal with Medi-Cal and Medicare, keep in touch with each patient's physician, update medication, and monitor patient compliance. I do all this in addition to changing dressings, filling insulin syringes, and providing emotional support. My patients range in age from thirty-five to ninety-three.

Although I do not have as many AIDS patients as I would like, the subject of mortality is always at front-and-center of my work. One of my former patients was Manuel Zarate, a blind, diabetic seventy-one-year-old man with renal failure. He got dialysis Mondays, Wednesdays, and Fridays; I saw him Tuesdays and Thursdays. The dialysis nurse had told me that Señor Zarate was on a tight fluid restriction, and he could drink no more than four glasses of water a day.

When I told Señor Zarate what the nurse had said, he got upset and complained, "They are depriving me of food and water!"

"I know this is hard for you," I said, "but this is the only thing we can do. Your wife will help."

"I don't want to do this anymore."

"What do you want to do?"

"I want to die."

I thought, "Oh, God!" Finally, I said, "Look, I can't understand fully how you feel. But I can tell you that I am here to help. Dialysis is keeping you alive. Medi-Cal is paying for it. And your family wants you to live."

He calmed down. When I left him, I was almost in tears. That is unusual, though. Generally, I leave my work behind. I do a bit of venting when I get home, but that's it.

(This patient finally decided that he could not go on with dialysis. His wife took him back to Mexico so he could die in his homeland. I got to see him before he left. It was sad to say goodbye, but I am consoled by the fact that he got his last wish—to die in Mexico.)

Sometimes I wonder if the whole Medicare structure will be bankrupt by the time I'm sixty-five. My tax dollars are paying for poor people like Señor Zarate to have health care. When I'm old and sick, who's going to pay for me? But if people need help, they should get it. To my way of thinking, it is immoral to let patients die if you can do something to save them.

Several weeks into my job at the VNA, I had a close call.

I have a patient named Maria Falcone. She is sixty-five, demented, and disoriented. She is also incontinent and requires an in-dwelling Foley catheter, used to drain urine from the bladder. I began seeing Mrs. Falcone every weekday in March 1995. One Friday, I did my usual checkups, didn't see anything wrong, and left. Another nurse saw her on Saturday. On Monday morning, Ms. Marshall, my supervisor, called me into her office.

"Did you know that Mrs. Falcone fell?" she asked.

"Her daughter didn't mention anything to me about a fall," I replied.

"She fell and fractured her arm. Didn't you notice anything?"

I said that Mrs. Falcone wears a long-sleeved nightgown and a robe. Furthermore, she's obese and sometimes it is hard to discern swelling in an overweight patient.

"They had to take her to the emergency room. The weekend nurse found her with an arm swollen to twice its normal size."

I thought, "Oh, no!"

I tried to defend myself. The truth is, Mrs. Falcone just looked heavy.

Then Ms. Marshall said, "Did you notice anything with the Foley catheter?"

Mrs. Falcone had been in the hospital for dehydration so I wasn't surprised to see that her urine output was low. I notified her doctor about the small amount of urine in the Foley bag, and he advised Mrs. Falcone to drink more fluids. He also said that if she didn't have more output by the next day, she would have to go to the emergency room. She ended up there anyway because of her arm.

While she was at the hospital, it was discovered that the Foley catheter had gotten clotted. I was stunned. I had taken the tubing apart and irrigated it with sterile water. The problem was, I had not documented my work. I figured I was only troubleshooting. Suddenly, I heard one of my instructors at Columbia saying, "If you don't document it, you didn't do it."

This poor woman was demented, swollen, and at risk for poisoning by her own urine. Luckily, her problems were caught in time. Now I am ultra-vigilant. Every time I see an elderly patient,

I ask, "Have you fallen recently?" And I write everything down. I love home health care and want to stay at this job forever. But I never stop feeling a little scared because I know I am always out in the field alone.

Rachel Rivera remains a home health-care nurse for the Visiting Nurse Association and Hospice of Northern California.

3

Desert Storm: All for One and One for All

NANCY JEAN MURRAY

My family has a history of performing military service. My mother was an army nurse during World War II. She met my father, a British naval officer, in Algeria. My uncle served in Korea; my brother and cousin went to Vietnam. We all believe that doing military duty is an honorable act, and I was eager to do my part. My first and only year as an active-duty army nurse turned out to be the highlight of my life.

After I graduated from the Medical College of Pennsylvania with a master's degree in anesthesia, I signed up for the Army Reserves. All my papers were in order, and I was ready to start basic training at Fort Dix. But four months into my anesthesia career, fate intervened to alter my plans: I got slapped with a group malpractice suit. The army refused to process my induction unless I cleared my name.

This is what happened. I was the nurse anesthetist for a prostate operation. The anesthesiologist needed a break, so I covered for him. On his way out of the operating room, he told me everything was fine. But as soon as he left, I heard the resident say that the patient was not doing well.

Under anesthesia or during TURP (trans-urethral resection prostate) surgery, a patient can overhydrate. This patient had absorbed fluid from the irrigation solution. His electrolytes were diluted, which meant that any number of his body's inorganic compounds—sodium, potassium, magnesium, calcium, chloride, and/or bicarbonate—were rendered ineffective and incapable of controlling internal fluid balance. He had a seizure and died on the operating table.

Water intoxication does not happen in two minutes, which is about how long I was in the OR. This problem had developed cumulatively over the course of about an hour and a half. But the anesthesiologist pointed the finger at me. Despite the aggravation I had to endure, the legal system ultimately vindicated me. The patient's doctors testified that they had told the anesthesiologist that the patient needed to "draw a sodium," or perform a test to determine how much anesthetic fluid the patient had absorbed. The anesthesiologist kept saying, "We'll do it in the recovery room." Well, the patient never made it there.

Five years down the road, I won a summary judgment, a ruling that cleared me of all culpability in the patient's death. Some people have the mistaken notion that a nurse cannot be named in a malpractice suit. Nurses have to understand that along with their expanded roles comes responsibility for outcomes. Believe me, if you are at the scene of an operation with a bad outcome, the burden is on *you* to clear your own name.

Once the court released me from the proceedings, the army accepted me. By March 1989, I was in uniform and spending one weekend a month at Fort Dix, New Jersey, administering anesthesia for hernia operations. It wasn't exactly extracting shrapnel, but I did end up meeting a lot of wonderful people.

But the whammy was coming, and it was Desert Storm.

In February 1990, I got the word to report for basic training. There was nothing in the news to indicate that the United States was gearing up for war anywhere in the world. I went off jauntily to Fort Sam Houston, Texas, believing that I was in for an adventure. Our commander asked, "If the U.S. declared war tomorrow, would you be willing to protect and defend your country?" I sat there thinking, "Oh, yeah, sure!" From my vantage point in New Jersey, I assumed that my seeing war anywhere was pretty remote. Still, I fully understood and accepted the possibility.

Then came August 1990. I was working as a freelance nurse anesthetist in the Poconos. I was watching TV in the hospital lounge when anchorman Dan Rather announced that Saddam Hussein had invaded Kuwait. I swear to God, I got a strange sensation in my stomach, and I thought, "This is more than a little ripple in history. Something big is going to happen. And it's going to happen to me." Sure enough, the Army told us, "Prepare yourselves."

I had my lawyer draw up a will. I gave her power of attorney to pay my bills while I was gone. Fortunately, I did not have to worry about leaving children behind. One of our female sergeants did. We were already in Saudi Arabia when she got a Red Cross message that her baby-sitter had upped and left the kids. Her seventeen-year-old daughter stepped into the breach and took care of the younger child.

I was mobilized as the anesthetist for the 718th Neurosurgical Detachment. The men and women of the 718th became my friends and family for the next seven months. We began our journey together at Fort Indiantown Gap near Carlisle, Pennsylvania, in November 1990, where we reported for two weeks of intensive training. For the first time in my life I held an M-16 in my hands. Outfitted in chemical gear, I got into a gas chamber to make sure my mask fit properly. I kind of laughed at all these preparations. I thought "What the hell have I gotten myself into?"

Time magazine ran pictures of military personnel headed for Saudi Arabia. They were waiting on long snaking lines beside airplanes. I ended up in one of those lines. I kept thinking, "What the hell have I done?" Eighteen hours after boarding my plane, I was in Dhahran in Saudi Arabia. My group stayed in the port of Dammam for two weeks while awaiting further orders.

Because we were in a detachment with a full-bird colonel as our commander, we thought, "We're in Fat City!" We figured we would land in a well-protected, fixed facility where the colonel could do neurosurgery. I remember asking an engineer in Dammam where the Twelfth Evac was going, because we were going with them. He walked over to a big map on the wall and asked, "What rank are you?" I told him I was a captain. He said, "All right, Captain. This is where you're going." He stretched his arm way up high and pointed to a place on the map forty miles south of the Iraqi border.

"Where are the troops that are going to protect us?" I asked.

He reached down about as low as he could, near his knee, and said, "The troops will be here for six weeks."

All I could think was, "Oh, my God, we're in trouble."

That was a bad time for me. When I wanted explanations, I was told, "You don't need to know." It began to dawn on me that I, as an individual, had no value. My group and I had a job to do: We were to set up support services for American troops. I, Nancy Jean Murray, could be sacrificed for a greater cause. In my first couple of days in-country, I was grieving the loss of myself as an individual. I knew that if this hospital got blown up, the military would consider its destruction acceptable. And if Saddam's Republican Guard attacked us, *I*, a five-foot-one-inch, thirty-six-year-old woman from Pine Beach, New Jersey, would have to fight to save myself and my colleagues.

But that's war, and that's what we all had to learn in those first few days. Once we learned this fact, we handled our situation with solidarity and laughter. It was an important change of attitude, and one that actually helped us *enjoy* ourselves.

Before I was mobilized, my mother, the World War II army nurse, said, "The army takes good care of you. They make wonderful food. They give you hot showers. And they always deliver the mail."

Well, we got some prepared foods, but most often we got MREs, which are "Meals Ready to Eat" that come in a plastic pouch. MREs were designed to feed a twenty-year-old boy with a sixty-pound pack on his back. They are loaded with calories, but plenty of walking around the base everyday kept the weight off me. At first, we did not have hot water for showers or for food. We heated up those delectable MREs on the engine block of our truck. This was not fun. Because we were reservists, the army initially did not supply us with electricity or kerosene, and it was cold in the desert at night. The active-duty hospital staff, on the other hand, got by completely on federal funding and did not seriously lack any amenities. After a few days, our blessed colonel managed to get us some private funding for a generator. I could even run my blow-dryer on it. We had the best hair in the Gulf.

Setting up the evacuation hospital was less frustrating. The army said, "Colonel, what do you need to begin work?" The colonel said he would need about $200,000 worth of instruments, plus a CT scanner. We received the instruments from Germany, and some two weeks later a helicopter arrived with the CT scanner housed in an air-conditioned container. We didn't have X-ray film at the time, so we CT-scanned simple fractures.

The hospital was a DEP-MEDS transportable modular unit

that consisted of tentage for wards and four categories of expandable containers for the lab, X-ray equipment, operating rooms, and pharmacy. Getting the hospital ready, however, did little to hide the bleakness of our situation. We were in the desert on December 21 with no prospect of receiving mail or presents. It was a lonely, scary time as we waited for the war to begin.

I was in the hospital on the night of January 17, 1991, when somebody came through screaming that we had to get into our chemical weapons gear. The United States had just bombed Baghdad. I began shaking. That night, we heard our tanks and armored vehicles off in the distance. My only solace was that we were to get into our suits but not the headgear. I wasn't sure exactly why we could take halfway measures, but I figured this meant that there were no scud missiles in the air—a good sign.

Every time our satellites picked up a scud launch in Iraq, everyone put on chemical weapons gear, including the headgear. At one point in the operating room, I was entirely suited up. I had to feel pulses and watch monitors because I couldn't hear a thing with that stuff on. The patient was the safest person in the hospital. He or she breathed filtered oxygen, nitrous oxide, and anesthetic gases. And much of the time, the patient was peacefully asleep and unaware that a war was in progress.

We had five different waves of patients. The first had developed their medical problems before the war started, mostly appendicitis, knee injuries, and injuries sustained in motor vehicle accidents. My first case was an eighteen-year-old boy with a perirectal abscess. He had been sitting in a tank for four months waiting for the war to start. He got dirty!

The second wave of patients had battle injuries. I worked on a tanker whose tank had gotten hit. He had tried to rescue his buddies from a burning tank, but he was the only one to escape. A young kid.

Next came the prisoners of war. These people struck me as ordinary citizens sent to the front as cannon fodder. The Republican Guard, Saddam's elite, loyal forces, were mean guys, but these POWS were ordinary citizens. Some of them were still carrying the groceries they had bought before they were forcibly inducted into military service. More than a few were highly educated. One was a cardiac surgeon. Another was a dentist. They arrived at the evac hospital starved and emaciated with no blankets or clothing. They told us, "We love Boosh!" Who knows? When they were repatriated, they may have said, "We love Saddam!"

The fourth wave of patients were mostly southern Shiite women and children. Their husbands had rebelled against Saddam in the vain hope of establishing a less dictatorial government. Saddam sent his Republican Guard to the towns south of Basra, turned his artillery on the people, and leveled the towns. Most of the men were dead. The women and children had the worst injuries of all the people we saw. One seven-year-old girl had been hit in the thigh with a missile; seven inches of her femur bone were missing. Another little girl had shrapnel in her eye. Her father asked the colonel if he could give her a fake eye. The colonel had to explain that although the technology for a good prosthesis existed, it was doubtful that we could get one before he and his daughter were repatriated. The fact is, we couldn't save every person. We couldn't make everything right. We could only do what we could do. So right now there is a young girl walking around Iraq with no eye. In her society, this can mean a dubious future as far as marriage is concerned.

One woman came to us with an eighteen-day-old baby who had spina bifida. This is a birth defect in which there is an opening in the spinal cord filled with dysfunctional nerves and spinal fluid. Usually, in a nontechnological society, the prognosis for a child with spina bifida is poor: The blister on the spinal cord bursts;

the child gets meningitis and dies. Through a Kuwaiti interpreter, the mother told us that she had gone into a hospital near Basra to have her baby. She delivered twins, a boy and a girl. When her husband came to visit, one of the hospital personnel recognized him as one of the rebels. The Republican Guard killed him and the newborn boy. They threw the mother and sick baby girl into the street. She saw an American helicopter and flagged it down. About all we could do for the child was to close the defect and shunt the brain so that the cerebrospinal fluid wouldn't accumulate in the cranium and cause a condition known as hydrocephalus. I was particularly proud of that surgery.

I would go into the wards and talk to the Iraqis. They were all literate, middle-class people who never thought something like this could happen to them.

The fifth wave of patients had injuries stemming from ordnance accidents. These included Americans, Iraqi children, and shepherds who had gone roaming around the desert, picking up or stepping on our unexploded cluster bomblets. I have spent many a night wondering why the army didn't emphasize the danger of ordnance, especially to those of us who had little military experience. I was luckier than most because my brother, who had been in Vietnam, wrote me letters instructing me not to touch *anything*. Ordnance comes in all different colors, shapes, and sizes and looks very interesting. People picked up the bomblets and played with them—until the bomblets blew up in their faces. The resulting injuries and deaths were sad and unnecessary. Evidently, trophy hunting always has been a problem in wars.

The day Saddam bombed Israel, I was sitting at a table in our tent. I thought, "Okay, we're toast." I said to myself, "This is going to turn ugly; this desert will become one great glass slag. And I'm going to have a front-row seat." People like to think that

Desert Storm was a big computer game. It wasn't. Especially if you were there.

Several months after I came back to the United States, I showed my Desert Storm photographs at a party. One of the guests was an attorney's wife. She didn't work outside the home, and her husband's money cushioned her from the dark exigencies of life. She took a look at the picture of the little girl with no eye and then slammed the photo album shut. The woman cried out, "Why are you showing us these pictures? They are disgusting!"

I studied the woman's blank face and said, "It was a war. It wasn't fun." She was offended that I would disturb her little New Jersey utopia. Well, life ain't that great all the time.

I have several souvenirs from Desert Storm. One is a right-arm patch, which indicates that you have served in a battle zone. It's really odd that there are career-army guys who never saw battle, and here I am, a *nurse*, with this highly coveted patch.

Another item is the *Prayer Warriors Pocket New Testament*, compliments of the U.S. Army. Ironically, it seems to indicate a religious justification for war and all that goes along with it.

I joined the Army Reserves willingly and knowingly, fully aware of what could happen. It was an honor to be in the army. It was an honor to go to the Gulf and work side by side with army medical personnel. And it was a particular honor to help care for U.S. soldiers in Desert Storm, which has become an important part of my personal history.

Nancy Jean Murray is a freelance nurse anesthetist in New Jersey.

4

Gung Ho About Being a Nurse

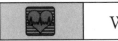 WARREN KEOGH

My first job in health care was as a psychiatric technician at St. Vincent's Hospital in Harrison, New York. We techs often felt that the nurses just sat around in the nurses' station while we did all the work. I told the nurses that if I were a nurse, I would never sit behind a desk jawboning my time away. They idn't believe me. My supervisor said, "Prove them wrong."

So, five years later, here I am: I work as a staff nurse at Phelps Memorial Hospital in Tarrytown, New York, and you will *never* find me sitting behind a desk.

Florence Nightingale may have been a great crusader for public-health nursing and aseptic technique, but in many ways, her day of lording it over the patient is over. Today patients have more input into their own care, and if you want to be a good staff nurse, it's important that you sit down and listen to them. A lot of the time, a patient will reveal something important to a nurse that he or she would be uncomfortable telling a doctor. In fact, a good nurse can anticipate a patient's concerns. Some of my patients, for example, come to the hospital for chemotherapy or radiation treatments month after month, always alone, without any family or friends for moral support. With those patients it is crucial that you sit down and say, "Hey, what have you been doing in the last few weeks since I saw you?" I care not only about their medical regimen but also about their social and psychological life.

In nursing school, my instructors drilled one simple but essential fact into my head: The nurse is an agent for change. I take this to mean that the nurse can make or break the quality of health care. I work in a small community hospital. I am in this profession because I love patient care and to make the patients feel better. I could come to work like a mopey downer, but what good would that do anyone? If I've got worries of my own, I leave them at home.

I had this zealous attitude about patient care even as a student in nursing school. Any time I sensed a crisis in the hospital, I wanted to be at the scene. Of course, students are not allowed to intervene in any kind of emergency care, but I still wanted to observe. Whenever a nurse called a code, I wanted to watch. This may be why I felt equal to the task in the beginning of my career when I called my first code.

It was room 208. Another nurse and I were helping a female patient walk from the bathroom back to her bed. All of a sudden, the patient turned gray and hit the floor. We took her blood pressure and detected no pulse. I looked at the nurse; she looked at me. We started performing CPR and called a code. The ICU nurses and doctors rushed in and took over. The patient had a pulmonary embolism—the blockage of a blood vessel in the lung—and, surprisingly, she survived.

One of my most rewarding experiences in my first year was actually sad. An elderly patient—I'll call him Mr. Mitchell—was a Do Not Resuscitate; that is, he wanted no heroic measures taken to keep him alive. I was in the room holding his hand when he passed away. Soon Mr. Mitchell's daughter came to visit and found him dead. She was upset and wanted to know the details of her father's passing. I told her that he appeared to be comfortable and that he did not die alone; I had been there with him to the last. The woman was grateful to me for my compassion and broke down in tears. It was a sad moment, but that's when I felt gung ho about being a nurse. I had treated this man and his daughter the way I myself would want to be treated in the same situation.

My first year as a nurse was great because I had a wonderful mentor, Lois Becker (not her real name), who dragged me into every new situation. One day she wanted me to wrap the body of a patient who had just died. I said, "I don't think I can do this," but Lois grabbed me by the collar and said, "Come on!" This may sound macabre, but it was a very nice experience. Lois taught me not only the how-to of that task but also the respectful mind-set that you must bring to it.

Eventually, one of my long-term patients, whom I'll call Mrs. Cristenzio, passed away. I would not let General Service, the department responsible for taking the body to the morgue, carry her away. I had known this woman for a couple of years and could not stand to see her heaved onto a table like a side of beef. Another colleague and I treated Mrs. Cristenzio with kid gloves and personally escorted her to the morgue.

I learned in nursing school that even an unconscious patient can hear you. That's why you have to treat the patient with respect even before he or she wakes up. I always speak to my patients, alive or dead, as if they can hear me. I am not a religious man, but I cannot help but think that there is something beyond our present existence; I feel it incumbent on me to show respect to those who have moved on to the next plane.

My dad once commented that I must be immune to death because I am a nurse. I realize that in my daily brush with life and death, I may appear to face death coldly, but this is not an accurate description of my state of mind. As a nurse, I have learned to "look through" death. I do not believe it is the be-all and end-all of human existence. I suppose I am like Forrest Gump when he says, "Death is a part of life."

This sums up my philosophical outlook on death, but, I can assure you, I never want a patient to pass on to another world without getting a fair shot at this one. For example, I was worried sick after I mistakenly administered digoxin, a cardiovascular drug, to the wrong patient. I took the patient's pulse and listened to his heart for a minute, as hospital policy mandates. The patient had a high heart rate so I gave him the digoxin. The problem was, I had deviated from standard operating procedure by neglecting to look at the patient's name band. That's something a nurse has to do automatically.

Almost immediately I realized my mistake. I told my boss. We listened to the patient's heart rate. It started to drop! I was freaked out. I kept thinking, "I killed this guy. He had no reason to die, and I killed him."

The cardiologist came into the room. Standing next to him, I thought I was going to faint. Finally, the doctor said, "The problem here is that this patient needs digoxin."

I blurted out, "My God! I just gave it to him by accident."

The cardiologist said, "Give him another dose!"

Occasionally, I will wake up in the middle of the night from a "nursemare," as we nurses at Phelps call it. A nursemare is a temporary state of panic that a nurse has when he or she wakes up at 2:00 A.M. and resists the impulse to call the hospital and say, "Did I give Mrs. Huntington her medication? Did I forget to drain the fluid from Mr. Ostrow's chest?" Nurses are prone to nursemares because they know that one inadvertent error can spell the difference between a patient's life and death.

Strangely enough, I worry much less about my own welfare. If an AIDS patient of mine started bleeding, I know I would do whatever it took to stop the bleeding. If I were walking down the street and saw a guy collapse on the corner, I would not hesitate to give him mouth-to-mouth resuscitation. I wouldn't care if the guy was puking, bleeding, or having a seizure. I realize that doing this might increase my risk of contracting the HIV virus, but I've come to believe that God is watching over me.

Warren Keogh, an oncology nurse at Phelps Memorial Hospital in Tarrytown, New York, is pursuing a master's degree in hospital administration.

5

Giving Kids Hope: The Mission of Child Psychiatric Nursing

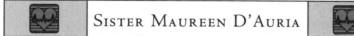

SISTER MAUREEN D'AURIA

When I entered the Catholic Congregation of the Sisters of St. Joseph of Peace, I wanted to become a nurse. At first this order directed me to teach primary and secondary school and to obtain a baccalaureate degree in biology. Both endeavors ultimately provided a solid foundation for nursing, which I was able to pursue at the Columbia-Presbyterian School of Nursing in 1970. I would have served in whatever mission the congregation deemed right, but I have always been grateful for the mutual discernment that led me to nursing. I know now that my path, beginning with my young students, was a journey better than anything I could have designed for myself.

My first job as a nurse was at Columbia's Babies Hospital. Usually, one L.P.N., an aide, and I cared for thirty-six children, most of them victims of cancer or other devastating diseases. My colleagues were supportive, and I was fortunate to have a mentor who spent most of her career working with grief-stricken families. She led support groups in which we could ventilate our anxieties about the children, and about their parents, some of whom were wrestling with drug addiction and alcoholism.

One of my first patients was a four-year-old boy named David Benton. When I was still a nursing student, he was diagnosed with leukemia. His parents' marriage was shaky, and David's illness destabilized it further. The Bentons got divorced. David himself was a wise child. He did not want to die, and yet, as he approached his seventh birthday, he started making provisions for his death. (I have seen many dying children do this. They will say, "I want my sister to have this doll." Or, "It's time for me to put on my new pajamas," meaning, "I want to be buried in these clothes." Frequently, a child near death holds on until the parents visit one last time. As soon as they leave, the child passes on to the next world.) David died at 5:00 A.M. with his mother at his bedside. I confess, I was relieved when he left us because he had suffered so much.

I respected my mentor's attitude about dying. She said that it was our job to give the kids hope. She encouraged us not to fixate on the child's symptoms, but rather, to see the child as a human being who had symptoms of a particular disease. She would never let a terminally ill child languish all day in his pajamas. In her characteristically kind manner, she would say, "Would you like me to help you put your clothes on?" Her implicit message was, "I'm not giving up on you."

Virgin Campbell was another child from the early days of my career. She was thirteen years old and seven months pregnant. The "father" was a sixty-year-old man who had also raped two other young girls. He used his young niece as a pimp. Virgin's mother was heartbroken. She herself was a woman in her thirties with three other children. The beautiful part of this story is that Virgin's family helped raise the child while Virgin went back to school and got her high school diploma.

Four years later I ran into a girl in East Harlem who looked at me and said, "Maureen, remember me? I'm Virgin." I hadn't recognized her. She was now seventeen, a high school graduate, and the mother of a four-year-old child. Although her life was full of hardship, Virgin, with the help of her family, was on a better, if not perfect, path. I felt privileged to share in Virgin's life, and in the lives of others who, like Virgin, invited me into their family circle, no matter how broken it may have been.

Eventually, I became a clinical specialist in child psychiatric nursing. In my first year as a visiting nurse, I was on my way to see a family in East Harlem when it dawned on me that I was in dangerous territory. Instead of feeling afraid, however, I was visited by a sense of peace, as if I were not walking alone. I understood that fear would inhibit my work, so I simply let it go. Now my real work as a nurse and as a sister of peace could begin.

I used to go into people's homes to do family therapy. Nobody knew I was a sister. One time, in fact, a man named José Vargas confided in me that he could not talk to a particular nurse because she was a sister. He proceeded to unburden himself to me because, as he said, I, a "plain old nurse," understood. José told me that he had dealt drugs and used them, and now had AIDS. His wife, he said, was in jail for armed robbery. José used to say, "Poor people need a revolution so they don't have to resort to criminal activity, like dealing drugs, to survive." He was perceptive about the relationship between poor, broken families and antisocial behavior. I thought him a wonderful man, especially because he, and his wife, too, loved their young son. Although they themselves had engaged in criminal behavior, they strove to protect their child from going down the wrong path. José was a good man, and I considered him a gift in my life. I spoke at his funeral when he died—and so did the other sister whom he couldn't talk to.

I learned early in my career that in New York City, people's basic human needs are frequently not met. You see this plainly in the health-care arena where poor people do not get continuity of care. Because they rarely have a personal doctor, they wait until their symptoms turn into a full-blown crisis before seeking help. For example, one of my patients, whom I'll call Alvinia New-combe, was a seven-year-old girl with sickle cell anemia. Her grandmother, her sole caretaker, had let the disease progress for so long without observation or treatment that Alvinia could no longer walk. Like many poor patients, Alvinia ended up in a hos-pital emergency room, where an anonymous doctor and other health-care providers touched and prodded and probed. Before she was transferred to a children's rehab hospital, I said to her, "I hope that when you come back to visit, you'll walk here on your own two feet." In one of those extraordinary professions of faith, Alvinia said, "Maureen, I'm not going to walk. I'm going to dance." And she did!

For every Alvinia, however, there are many more people who cannot even tell you the name of the doctor, nurse, or social worker they have seen. And many times, the doctor does not know the patient's name. It's often an inhuman system for both patient and health-care provider. In poor urban communities, some peo-ple are resigned to the fact that just about anybody in the health-care field has a right to touch them, and that they themselves cannot be involved in their own care.

As a visiting nurse, I had to win my patients' trust. Sometimes I had to visit a home several times before the people inside would let me in. I think they wanted to be sure I was committed to them. Once inside, I could take in their financial circumstances at a glance. Perhaps they had a TV. Toys were scarce because they cost a lot of money, and a bike rarely lasted more than a few weeks; bikes were easy prey for thieves.

I would do play therapy with the children. Just as important, though, I had to parent the parents. When parents are struggling to meet basic human needs, they don't have much energy left over to spend time with their children. The people I saw worried constantly about getting money, paying rent, and buying food. Poverty of spirit and economics are intertwined and intergenerational: Their own parents had been in the same boat. Given such stressful circumstances, child abuse was always a possibility in these homes. Anticipating it, I would give the mothers puppets and crayons and let them dramatize their anxieties. They thought this was fun. *Nobody had ever played with them like this before.* How can people be creative with their own children when the stress of survival is their daily plight?

I was careful not to be negative or overbearing with my patients. Instead of saying, "You watch too much TV," or, "You don't have any marketable skills," I would enlist them in the creation of their own care plan. That is really what psychiatric nursing is about: getting the *patient* to figure out how to improve his or her own life.

Whenever I got frustrated by the degradation in my patients' lives, I thought back to a statement that one of my Catholic sisters made: "Change comes only from the grass roots, and that's *you.*" José, the man who died of AIDS, understood this too. My mission as a nurse, and as a sister, is to encourage people to embrace their human rights for good health care, a decent education, and a safe place to live.

I do not have to go to farflung places like Bangladesh or Rwanda to "save" bodies and souls. The people who need me are here in East Harlem, Newark, and Jersey City. I need them too.

Sister Maureen D'Auria is a clinical specialist in psychiatric nursing with the York Street Project in Jersey City, New Jersey.

6

Have We Created a Medical Monster?

 E L A I N E   B R E N N A N

Forty-one ailing veterans made up my first patient load. In the course of eight hours, I had to give each one of them multiple medications. I worked on a medical floor at Manhattan's Veterans Administration Hospital and took care of men who had fought in World War I, World War II, and Korea. Twenty or thirty years of hard drinking had turned the livers of many of them to Jello, and now they needed round-the-clock care.

I was twenty-one years old and a recent graduate of the Seton Hall University School of Nursing in South Orange, New Jersey. Seton Hall was one of the few four-year baccalaureate nursing programs in the late 1950s, and because we students were viewed as pioneers, our instructors treated us like little princesses. My education, along with my own desire to care for people in need, emboldened me to take on any nursing task, no matter how formidable. I was also motivated by the fact that nursing was a line of work in which you could see the results of your labors. You established a relationship with your patient. You watched him get better or helped make his death less painful. At the end of the day, you knew you had done worthwhile work.

In the beginning of my seventeen-year tenure at the VA Hospital, I worked the evening shift. My first night on duty, it took me forever to do my rounds. One hour passed, two, three. I made mincing headway. In the blink of an eye, it was time to get the men ready for bed. I looked down the hall and saw Flossie Corcoran, a nursing attendant who had worked at the Veterans Hospital for a million years and knew all the ropes.

Flossie had pulled her linen-and-lotions cart up to the nurses' station. She stood there watching me, one hand under her elbow and the other cupping her chin. I knew she wanted to see me, but I couldn't move. I was buried under the weight of my workload and petrified to make a mistake. Flossie Corcoran crooked her index finger at me. I stopped dispensing meds and walked over to her cart.

"What's up?" I asked.

Firmly, Flossie said, "Let's go." This kindhearted woman understood that I was in a panic. She walked beside me, saying, "This is the routine. Here is what you have to do. . . ." I am eternally grateful to her for getting me through that night, and others like it.

Flossie's help notwithstanding, I did not become a good nurse overnight. One of my first patients was a young Italian man with leukemia. He and his girlfriend had wonderful personalities, and the nurses became attached to both of them. The couple decided to get married, but he was too sick to leave the hospital. The nurses arranged for the chaplain to come to the patient's bedside and perform the ceremony. They also brought flowers and canapés and had a little reception for the two of them.

One day shortly after the ceremony, this lovely man went into shock. His spleen had ruptured. He was dying! I absolutely fell apart. I didn't know what to do for him. I started to cry.

The patient saw how upset I was. He reached his hand out to me and said, "Take it easy. Everything will be all right." I could not believe I had lost control. The patient had to calm *me* down.

That taught me an important lesson about professionalism. The nurse has a specific role in the care of patients, and she or he has to play it. There is something wrong with a nurse who cannot connect to a suffering human being; still, the nurse must also assume a measure of emotional distance.

Working on a ward full of grizzled veterans, I had many opportunities to toughen up. One of my "teachers" was a cranky old guy named Eugene Stulac. Like a lot of the vets, Eugene had cirrhosis of the liver. He reminded me a little of my grandpa, so I got attached to him too. Eugene used to regale me with all his old army stories.

One morning, as I began my shift, Denise Johns, the night nurse, gave me a rundown on all my patients. Denise got to Eugene's name and said, "Poor old Eugene. He's really failing fast. He's so weak he can't even close his mouth."

I was stunned. "Really!" I said. "He didn't seem so bad yesterday."

"Yeah, well, his mouth is just hanging open," Denise said.

When Denise finished giving me the night's report, I went into Eugene's room. Sure enough, Eugene's mouth was hanging open. He was just waking up, and I asked him, "Eugene, how ya doing?"

All he could say was: "Aah! Aah!"

"Eugene, what's the matter!"

Again: "Aah! Aah!"

Clearly, he wasn't weak, but something was wrong with his

mouth. I rushed into the doctor's office. "Something's wrong with Eugene!" I shouted. "I can't figure out what's going on."

The doctor examined Eugene and discovered that the old guy had dislocated his jaw by yawning. Well, I couldn't help but laugh to myself. We put an ace bandage around Eugene's head so that the jaw could heal. Eight hours later Denise came back on duty. She remarked how "poor Eugene" looked weaker than ever with the bandage on. Denise Johns may have been a seasoned army nurse, but she sure missed the boat on that one!

In my first year out of nursing school, the Veterans Hospital opened its first intensive care unit. I applied to work there because I thought it would be a challenge. It was. The unit had twelve beds and four heart monitors. We nurses thought that was hot stuff. Of course, when we got our first cardiac patient, we had no idea what the monitor was saying. The cardiologist came in and drew a couple of pictures on a piece of paper. "This is a P-wave," he said. "That's when the atrium contracts." He drew a vertical line and said, "That's QRS. That's when the ventricle contracts. This bump is when they both rest. If anything changes, call me." Thus, my first crash course in critical care.

Some of my first ICU patients had severe lung disease and were managed in the iron lungs. One day during my shift, a surgeon came in to do an emergency tracheotomy, which meant cutting into a patient's windpipe. As he opened the iron lung, he ordered me to get a sponge.

I ran to the sink and saw a giant sponge stuck through with used syringe needles. I called back to the doctor, "How big do you want it?"

He measured off about four inches with his hands. I took this ordinary sink sponge and cut it to his specifications.

When I handed the doctor the sponge, he looked at me as if I had lost my mind. In his lexicon, *sponge* meant a sterile gauze pad, not a kitchen sponge. Now Denise Johns wasn't alone in the "Department of Embarrassing Bloopers!"

As part of our ICU training, we nurses studied heart function in a dog lab. The researchers would shock a dog's heart to provoke cardiac arrhythmia, a disturbance in the rhythm of the heartbeat. They shocked it again to provoke normal heart rhythm. We had an extensive training program in cardiac resuscitation, which included massaging the dog's heart with our hands.

Soon after my experience in the dog lab, the doctors brought a cardiac patient into the ICU. Immediately, the patient had a heart attack. In one second, he was dead. We shocked him, and just like that, he woke up and began talking as if nothing had happened. When I first became a nurse, I knew I would see some gruesome and astonishing sights, but I never imagined seeing a dead man brought back to life. Fitzsimmons was his name. I'll never forget him. Bed 4.

Sometimes, I think, we have become all too good at "waking the dead." The Korean War vets I saw had not suffered life-threatening wounds; by the time they arrived at the VA Hospital, their vital signs were stabilized and their wounds had begun to heal. The mortally wounded died on Korean soil. By the first years of the Vietnam War, however, science had perfected the art of medical transport and emergency treatment. Now medics treated soldiers on-site quickly. As a result, they were able to keep more severely injured soldiers alive, so men arrived at the VA hospital with holes in their heads, half their bodies blown off, and an addiction to drugs. Some of these guys did not want to be kept alive.

My job was to keep them alive, just as I had kept Eugene Stulac alive. Before the Vietnam War, nursing care and medicine had been pretty straightforward. Gravely wounded people used to die, but advances in trauma care have decreased mortality rates—and created a lot of the ethical dilemmas that confront us today.

Elaine Brennan graduated from Seton Hall University School of Nursing. She held a variety of clinical roles in nursing for twenty years and is now vice president of operations at Montefiore Medical Center in Bronx, New York.

7

A Pediatric Nurse Learns the Ropes

 LEAH HARRISON

On July 6, 1968, I arrived at Montefiore Medical Center with bright red ribbons in my hair. I was twenty years old, the holder of an associate degree from Pace University in Westchester County, New York, and an idealist bent on saving the lives of sick children. I thought my red ribbons would put my little patients at ease. After a couple days in Pediatrics, my supervisor informed me that ribbons were not part of a nurse's uniform. Regardless of whether they had appealed to the children, my ribbons obviously had *not* put the institution at ease.

My first job was in Pediatrics on the night shift. When the head nurse went out to eat dinner, I remained alone on the floor with only one nurse's aide. I felt an indescribable responsibility for the safety of the children. I listened to every creaking noise and anticipated the worst.

At one in the morning, I heard the elevator door open. A middle-aged gentleman came into view. As he approached the nurses' station, I stood up with great authority and announced, "You don't belong here! It is one o'clock in the morning, and unless you have a very good reason to be here, you must leave immediately. If you don't, I'm calling Security!"

My midnight interloper was Dr. Martin Cherkasky, then the president of Montefiore Medical Center. I had never met him, and he wasn't wearing his ID. I had tried to chase the president of Montefiore off the unit! Whenever I see him, I think of this funny incident.

In Pediatrics, our saddest cases were the kids with cancer. One little boy had Wilms' tumor, a form of cancer that grows on the kidney and abdomen. (Twenty-five years ago, Wilms' tumor was a death sentence. Today we have chemotherapeutic agents to fight it, and many kids survive.)

Several months into my job, a five-year-old black boy came into our ward. His father had pushed him out a window, and now the child was paralyzed from the waist down. For days he cried because he wanted his father. Nobody, not the nurses, the doctors, or the social workers, could console him. I was so perplexed. How could he still love his father after what his father had done to him?

As I began working with more abused children, I came to see that abuse alone does not make a child hate his or her parents. No matter how much the parents beat the child, they are still the child's parents, and the child loves them. Even if that little boy hated his father for what he had done, a voice inside him said, "If I don't love my daddy, who's going to love me?"

I was barely twenty-two when I realized that in order to "climb the ladder of success," I had to have advanced degrees. Montefiore paid part of my tuition for my bachelor's degree. After a while I wanted to become a nurse practitioner. I went back for a master's, and Montefiore paid half of that too.

While I was attending school for my master's degree, my husband encouraged me to go to medical school. His reasoning was, "If you're going to put in time at school, why not become a pediatrician? As a nurse, you will never be number one."

I thought about that. I concluded that I like the nursing focus more than medicine. As a nurse practitioner, I would expand my nursing role to include diagnosis and treatment. I could even write prescriptions. But for me, delivering health care was not just a matter of wielding more and more authority. I felt that my nursing experience and holistic philosophy had helped kids get better services. If I went to medical school, I was afraid I would become like some pediatricians who don't go all out for their patients. I did not want that to happen to me, so I vetoed medical school.

The only negative about being a nurse is that you don't have the clout a physician has. For the most part, people listen to a doctor before they listen to a nurse. Yet nursing is the only profession whose holistic philosophy mandates that you look at a person as one integrated human being, not simply as various organic systems. This is what makes the profession unique.

Leah Harrison was Nurse of Distinction for New York State in 1993. She is the associate director of the Child Protection Center for Montefiore Medical Center in Bronx, New York.

8

A Visiting Nurse
Confronts the Down
and Out

 PHYLLIS NEWTON

For you to understand why I wanted to work in the South Bronx, I have to talk first about my life as a daughter of Christian missionaries. I grew up in Sidon, Lebanon, where my Jewish mother, a convert to Christianity, ran a school for street children and my father did ministry work in the nearby villages. What with all the different ethnic and national groups in Sidon, life was tense. It might have been worse had our Palestinian neighbors known that my mother was Jewish. As it was, people once shot at us and threw stones several times as we walked down the street. A Jewish Christian in an Arab world does not have an easy fate. For as long as I can remember, danger has been a normal part of my life.

When I began working for the Visiting Nurse Service of New York in 1972, I understood that a threat to my personal safety would be a fact of life. During my tenure as a nurse in the East

Tremont section of the Bronx, some of our nurses had been raped. I myself was nearly attacked once.

I sensed somebody following me, and when I turned around to look, I saw him, a large man half a city block behind me. I was carrying my heavy black nursing bag, which I could swing in an emergency. Realistically speaking, though, I knew I was defenseless against a knife, the typical weapon of choice back then. Out of desperation, I rushed into the first building I could. Of course, I might have rushed into an even worse predicament, but, as in other times in my life, I was protected. I kept knocking on doors until finally someone let me in.

My patients were my reward. The most challenging were the Puerto Rican teenage girls who came to see me for drug counseling and sex education in lieu of going to reform school. They would strut into my storefront office, equipped with their chains and brass knuckles, hardened to any expression of human kindness. Most of them had run away from sexually and physically abusive parents or had been left homeless on the street. In nursing school, I had written my thesis on child abuse, so I was prepared for the worst. Already I had seen a child who had been dipped into boiling water at the age of two and had undergone innumerable skin grafts so he could walk again; he had lost the power of speech. Given the extent of drugs and violence in these girls' lives, none of them expected to survive their teenage years. In fact one of the girls was fourteen years old and had had a hysterectomy because while she was pregnant, she had been in a gang fight and somebody ripped her open.

To some extent, these girls could not make heads or tails out of me. They could not understand why I, a white person, cared about them. They also could not believe that, at twenty-three, I was still a virgin. I was moved by their curiosity. They had to ask me these intimate questions because they had no reliable mother figure in their lives. And they could not handle my love for them without questioning it.

I would have liked talking to the administrator of the Tremont district office about the misery I saw everywhere. Unfortunately, Tina Hendricks (not her real name) was an embittered woman in her late fifties, resentful of the nurses who had bachelor's degrees, and afraid of them too. I think she was instrumental in having me transferred from East Tremont to Lincoln Hospital in the southern section of the Bronx. To her mind, she had banished me to health-care Siberia. I, however, viewed my transfer as a blessing. I worked as a liaison between the hospital and the community, and gained entrée into the lives of people I would otherwise not have met.

My job was to visit the homes of patients who had been seen in Lincoln Hospital's emergency room or outpatient clinics. I followed up on children diagnosed with anemia, malnutrition, and lead poisoning.

I remember one two-and-a-half-year-old African-American boy who had lead poisoning. He lived with his mother and grandmother in a dirty, sparsely furnished apartment. What struck me the most about this family was the centrality of the color TV set in their lives. The adults would camp out in front of the TV while the child, malnourished and anemic, ate paint chips. This wasn't necessarily a case of neglect. The adults had no idea that eating paint chips was a health hazard. They figured this was just something kids did.

Another child, a five-year-old Puerto Rican boy, came into the clinic one day in a deranged state. He had just tried to kill his grandmother, whom he lived with, and he had also tried to slit his own wrists. I tried to calm him down by singing to him, and praying for him, but he would scream out these bizarre oaths at me in Spanish. The look in his eye was wild.

When I went into his home, I saw a roomful of objects used in Santeria rituals, things like voodoo dolls and goats' teeth. The grandmother practiced some sort of spiritism, and since she was the only person around, the little boy had absorbed her teachings. When I recommended that he be committed to a psychiatric institute for children, both the boy and the grandmother disappeared.

Another child was an in-patient in the pediatric unit because he had compulsively banged his head against the wall. Some very young children do bang their heads, but by the time they are two, they stop. This boy was three and a half. After he left the hospital, I followed up on him in his home. His living arrangements were awful. He slept on a cot in a hallway. The wall behind his cot was dented in and flaking from where he had banged his head. While visiting, I saw the child bang his head and gnash his teeth, so I knew that nobody was actually ramming him against the wall. He lived in this place with his single mom, her boyfriend, and three other siblings. My sense was that he was the family's escape valve for their frustrations. I recommended that he be placed in a foster home, but nobody would take him. In any case, the mother put up a lot of resistance and there was not enough evidence to justify forcibly removing him from her custody.

During my first year as a nurse, I witnessed other less abusive, albeit painful scenarios. Some of my first patients were immigrants from eastern Europe. They had some unusual traditions, such as swaddling their babies on a board. You could always identify an eastern European child by the flattened back of his or her head. In and of itself, this custom had no negative effect on the children. The real problem was in the way the mothers fed their newborns. As "modern" women, they were opposed to breast-feeding and fed the babies formula. But because the women couldn't read English, they didn't know they had to dilute the formula. The infants ended up getting diarrhea and upset stomachs. I often had to teach pediatric care by doing hands-on demonstrations and using sign language.

I saw a lot of elderly diabetic patients, many of them Jews from eastern Europe. They had moved to the Tremont section of the Bronx a generation before the influx of younger Hispanic and black people. These old orthodox Jews would stay holed up in their apartments, too frightened to go out on the street. One sweet old lady, a diabetic in her eighties, kept kosher and observed the Sabbath. On Saturdays, when I arrived to give her her insulin, I would light the fire to heat her water. Observant Jews do not turn on lights or make fire on the Sabbath, so I would do this for her. It was painful to see somebody as delightful as she cower in her little apartment in her own neighborhood.

My work in the South Bronx was a rich experience, yet overall, I found New York City oppressive. I dreaded the subway. During rush hour, I would be crushed up against fifty other people, all jockeying for their few inches of turf. As a young visiting nurse dressed in a blue uniform, I was a magnet for every masher who got next to me. I hated the constant struggle of having to keep the city's depravity at bay. One time a guy got into my building and exposed himself. The police didn't do a thing. This rampant assault on my soul and senses got to me, and I moved out to Seattle to be near my family.

Sometimes I am overwhelmed by the amount of need in the world. Only my faith that there is some divine purpose in our lives gives me the courage to help one person at a time. I keep praying and let God do the rest. After all, He's omnipresent. I'm not.

Phyllis Newton's most recent medical mission was in Kenya.

9

Sticks, Stones, and Broken Bones

NAOMI SHUSTER*

Every day I would come home from work and think, "I want to quit."

My day began on the orthopedics floor of a hospital I'll call it Sterling Hospital—in upstate New York. I was responsible for five to seven patients. Average age: eighty-five. Before I started working, I thought orthopedics consisted of broken hips and spinal deformities. But these patients also had liver failure, heart disease, cancer, or dementia. Their conditions were so complicated that I often suffered from an overwhelming sense of incompetence.

Nothing has frightened me more than the thought of having to call a code. (A code is called when a patient has experienced a life-threatening physical crisis. Medical staff are summoned, and they must act quickly to save the patient's life.) Such a situation forces you to ask yourself some taxing questions. Such as: Can I deal with a crisis? Would I recognize the signs of impending death? If

---

*This is a pseudonym.

the patient dies, is it my fault? If the patient's family is in the hospital, am I capable of telling them that their loved one has died?

It's weird. A patient can appear to be at death's door and then survive for months. One of my psychiatric patients was a woman in her eighties with advanced renal failure. She was hooked up to an IV and a catheter, which she kept pulling out. I don't think she wanted to die, not consciously anyway. She was just off her rocker. On the day she died, her family telephoned. They asked me if I thought this woman was going to die soon. That day the patient had been having delusions, a "normal" state of affairs for her. I mean, she was making inappropriate sexual comments to the doctors, as always, so I figured she was her usual self. I told the family, "Actually, I think she is stable." Two hours after my shift, she died.

I felt awful. A couple of nurses told me that patients frequently look better before they die. I don't know if that's true. But if I had told this particular family that the patient was near death, they could have come to the hospital to pay their final respects. Nowadays I avoid the trap of predicting death. I simply say, "We have no idea when somebody's time is up."

In addition to the psychological strain of working with dying patients, I have had to contend with the physical demands of my job. Many orthopedic patients have had total hip replacements. If they move their legs recklessly, they can pop their hip out. Then they have to have surgery again. To avoid the pain and expense of resetting a hip, the nurse puts pillows between the patient's legs and then places the patient in another position. I cannot turn a patient by myself, so I have to wait for somebody to help me. Because of staffing cutbacks, the poor patient has to wait a long time. And teaching patients how to avoid popping a hip is often impossible because a lot of them are senile.

Nurses always talk about the procedures they hate. In general, I can help patients to the bathroom without feeling revolted. But when I was pregnant, my sense of smell became altogether too sophisticated. *C. dificile*, a bacterium that depresses the natural flora in the bowel, causes a vile odor, and smelling it made me retch.

Bedsores are also horrific. The wound can be necrotic, which means the affected tissue is dead, foul-smelling, and full of pus. A patient gets bedsores from lying around in bed and not moving. Incontinent patients are prone to bedsores because urine destroys the skin's integrity. I remember that one nursing student from the College of New Rochelle saw an egregiously bad bedsore and dropped out of her nursing program that day.

In the beginning, it is very hard to manage your time. You have seven patients, and you have to get them washed, medicated, or ready for surgery. You have patients that have to be discharged and others that have to be admitted. You have to hang containers of blood on IV poles, you have to change dressings. One day in my typical rush to appear efficient, I stuck myself with a needle.

The patient, an old man, had a heplock in his arm. This is basically a port into which the nurse hooks up IV tubing. In this case, I had hooked up the main line that contained saline solution and then piggybacked an antibiotic line into the saline. I stuck myself with the secondary tubing. Technically speaking, the antibiotic line did not come into contact with the man's body. But because the fluids all flow into each other, bacteria or viruses theoretically can travel up and down this tubing highway. My first thought was, "Okay, he's seventy-five years old and heterosexual." As we know, though, no demographic group is immune from acquiring HIV. I knew I had to be tested.

Fortunately, the man agreed to have his blood sampled. He was within his rights to refuse. We both tested negative. Even so, I was chastened. You can do one stupid thing in your mad dash to be efficient, and your life can be over.

Every now and then, I encounter an old competent person. That is a joy. I had one patient who, at 102, had tripped over a pebble while walking with her three sisters and had broken her hip. Mrs. Eve Masters was astute about the doctors, knew which ones she hated, which ones she liked, and which ones were prima donnas. We talked about her professional life when she was the principal of a public school in the Bronx. Her mind was as clear as a bell. After meeting her, I realized that losing your mind is a lot more degrading than experiencing the deterioration of your flesh.

In some cases, you can see the patient's character behind the body's devastation. Although one of my patients lost her speech after a stroke, I could see from her smile that she was a lovely woman. The patient's daughter loved her so much that she took care of her at home by herself.

In my eighth month as a nurse, I gave a blood transfusion to a woman who had congestive heart failure. The procedure demands as much art as science. In this woman's case, she could not handle a lot of fluids, and the blood had to enter her veins slowly. A lot of surgeons prefer a fast inflow; transfusing blood for longer than four hours can cause clotting. According to hospital policy, blood must infuse within a two- to four-hour time frame. Monitoring the influx of blood is not my favorite nursing task. You never know how the patient is going to respond. You have to monitor the transfusion all the time to watch for negative reactions. It's nerve-racking.

The patient's blood entered her bloodstream in about two

hours. After work, I got a call from a nurse, an L.P.N., who said, "Your patient went into distress." The next nurse had had to give her lasix, a diuretic, before giving her more blood. I mean, the patient didn't die. But this L.P.N. had taken it upon herself to tell me that I could have gotten into trouble for giving the blood too fast.

When I hung up the phone, my body was in a sweat. For moral support, I called a close friend with whom I had trained at McGill University. "Oh, my God!" I said. "I should have given her the blood more slowly!" My friend's husband, who is a doctor, got on the phone and said, "Look, she needed the blood. What difference does it make how fast you gave it to her? It was still too much fluid volume for her to handle. Two hours, three, four, would not have made a difference."

By the time I got off the phone, I was angry at the L.P.N. Who was she to be looking over my shoulder? In point of fact, my supervisor never even talked to me about this incident.

What I discovered is that your "fellow" nurses can really stick it to you in the back. Part of the problem lies in the hospital hierarchy. There are baccalaureate-trained nurses and L.P.N.s. There also are nurses with master's degrees. Each group seems to resent the others. As for the doctors, they can scream at you for nothing. Everything bad is the nurse's fault. I think a hysterical doctor forces a nurse to cover her own behind, and she is often ready to blame another nurse just to protect herself.

Add to this stew the racial tensions on the floor, and you have a less-than-perfect work environment. Racism in the hospital is not just a matter of blacks versus whites. It's more like a sea anemone, a creature with lots of tentacles branching out in many different directions. Several of my patients, for example, are racist and anti-Semitic. One former patient, Mrs. Alice Whitson, was a senile woman from an affluent family. With her everything was dirty

Jew this, dirty Jew that. She called her physician, Dr. Evan Thie-bold, a Jew even though he is every bit the WASP Mrs. Whitson is. I found it very hard to take care of this woman.

At the same time, I think that many nurses have a chip on their shoulder. Because racism is prevalent in the hospital, they often perceive racial conflict where it doesn't exist. It's a vicious cycle: The patient does not like being taken care of by a nurse with an attitude. So the patient requests another nurse. Then the patient looks like a racist whether he or she is one or not.

Now, if the head nurse at Sterling Hospital wasn't so incompe-tent, these racial tensions might not have the environment in which to flourish. But this nurse demonstrates the truth of the Peter Principle: She has been promoted to the level of her incom-petence. Her way of managing is to favor certain individuals. This does nothing to address tensions, racial or otherwise, that arise in the workplace. Pretending that racism doesn't exist doesn't make it go away. Many of the African-American nurses attribute her management style to racism. Really, she's plain old incompetent.

I have been working as a nurse for two years now. I am proud of myself for weathering all the storms—racial, interpersonal, and professional. In nursing school we learned that the hospital con-siders the nurse a liability for the first half-year; only after six months does the nurse become productive. I found that to be true. Because I was a Canadian-trained nurse, I had a hard time finding a job in the United States, and I knew I had to tough it out at Sterling whether I was happy or not. I did not have the economic latitude to quit.

I have learned that I do not have control over everything bad that happens. I certainly cannot control the condition in which the patient enters the hospital. Yet even now, when the telephone rings and it's someone from work, I think, "Oh, my God! I must have killed somebody!" It turns out that a nurse just wants to switch her schedule with me. Is that weird or what?

"Naomi Shuster" is a staff nurse at a hospital in New York State.

10

A Nurse Practitioner Abroad "Works Hard for the Money"

 LUCINDA WEBB

In the mid-1940s, my father was head of the International Refugee Organization in southern Europe. I would travel with him to displaced-persons camps in Austria, Italy, and the Balkans, and I would feel intrigued by the swarms of men, women, and children on their way to somewhere else. While my father tended to administrative matters, I would wander through the clinics, drawn to discover people through their illnesses and war wounds. When I returned to the United States in the 1950s, I planned on studying nursing and anthropology so that one day I could do international work as my father had done.

Life being unpredictable, I fell in love. I got my degree in anthropology, but instead of going to nursing school, I got married and had four children in the space of five and a half years. My ambition sat on the shelf until my husband and I decided to join the Peace Corps. We knew several people who had moved with their children to Africa and South America; peripatetic by nature and habit, we wanted to do the same. In 1971, I enrolled at the Columbia-Presbyterian School of Nursing in New York, and my husband prepared to leave the shipping business in order to get a graduate degree in math. Just as our plans fell into place, my husband died suddenly. He had hypertrophic cardiomyopathy, a congenital defect in which the heart walls thicken and obstruct blood flow into and out of the chambers. Just as suddenly, I was a widow with four children to support.

I was despondent, but Dean Helen Pettit at Columbia encouraged me to start nursing school on a part-time basis. I graduated in 1974 and was working as a nurse by May 1976.

My first stint as a nurse nearly turned me against the entire profession. I worked on a mixed ward at a Manhattan Catholic hospital—I'll call it St. Bartholomew's—as a staff nurse, doing everything from hanging IVs to baptizing miscarried fetuses. I treasure the few extraordinary events that happened on my watch: I saw a young boy come out of a hepatic (hepatitis-related) coma, which almost never happens past the eighteenth day. I became familiar with some taboos that Chinese women practice after childbirth (they don't shower for six weeks). And I met a patient who had given birth to a baby that had developed inside her abdominal cavity instead of her uterus. By some miracle, mother and child both lived and were in perfect health. This is the sort of rare phenomenon you read about in medical textbooks.

Overall, however, St. Bartholomew's was oppressive. Unlike Columbia, where a group of inter-disciplinary students used to meet to discuss ethical and social issues related to health care, St. Bartholomew's discouraged any sort of dialogue. The culture there was do-as-you're-told. It was also judgmental. When I arrived, I introduced myself as Ms. Webb, but my supervisor insisted on calling me Mrs. Webb, even though I wasn't married anymore. And when three nurses from India refused to take care of gays and sexually active, single heterosexual girls, the hospital did not reprimand them. My sense was that St. Bartholomew's also disapproved of the patients' behavior and let these nurses act unprofessionally. I had to get out of there, even if leaving meant I would never work as a nurse again.

My true nursing career began when I entered the adult nurse practitioner graduate program at Columbia. Before I was even out of the program, I asked Dr. Michael Stewart, chief of the Vanderbilt Clinic who had medical experience abroad, if he could find a summer position for me overseas. Dr. Stewart arranged for me to teach physical assessment skills with Project Hope in Egypt. I was ecstatic! With my four kids in tow, I went to Egypt, and after three weeks of sightseeing, I began teaching eight well-heeled, eloquent Egyptian women primary care at the High Institute of Nursing in Alexandria.

I learned as much from my students as they from me. About ten of us from the Project Hope staff went down to the City of the Dead in Cairo to witness the circumcisions of little girls and boys, all of them between the ages of six and eight. Needless to say, this was painful to watch. A big bruiser of a man held the children's legs apart so the children couldn't squirm. Amid a lot of weeping and howling, the deed was done.

In my view, circumcision for a six-year-old boy is painful, but for girls it is absolutely intolerable. The girls undergo a clitoridectomy, which entails the surgical excision of the clitoris. The clitoris is the trigger for female sexual response. Removing it makes arousal virtually impossible. Moreover, the little girls get lots of infections. Their mothers and aunts, who have also experienced the same mutilation, stand over the girls and shriek out an ululating lamentation. This is supposed to be an expression of joy, but, at the same time, it serves to drown out the little girls' cries. In parts of Egypt and the Sudan, "female circumcision"—actually genital mutilation—also involves removing the girls' labia. In other African countries, the circumcisers suture the vagina closed, leaving just enough of an opening for the menstrual flow. When the girls get married, they are unsutured.

While I was standing around, waiting for the so-called female circumcision to begin, my group of students asked the Egyptians to let me have a front-row seat. "She's a doctor," they said. "She does this in her country, and she has to see how you do it here." The Egyptians brought me into their inner circle.

It was terrifying. After they finished with one child, they asked me to show them my technique. I said I could do nothing to improve on anything they did. Their mutilation was perfect.

Back in the classroom, I asked, "If any of you had daughters, would you have them circumcised?" Some said they would rather leave the country than subject their daughters to this "barbaric" practice. Some said they thought female circumcision terrible, yet family pressure would compel them to have it done. As a cultural outsider, I could not probe into my students' personal lives. In any case, nobody would admit to having been circumcised herself. I suspect many of them had been.

I returned to Columbia and got my nurse practitioner degree. Toward the end of that year, 1979, Pol Pot invaded Cambodia. Almost immediately, the international community organized medical teams to take care of the thousands of Cambodian refugees streaming across the border to Thailand. I felt an incredible pull to get over there and begin my work as a nurse practitioner. By now all my children were either in college or in the last year of high school, and I knew that for a few months they could manage without me. I applied to the International Red Cross and learned that it was not accepting any Americans.

I was depressed. I had heard that nurses from New Zealand and Australia were flying to Bangkok and hitching onto medical teams from there. I could not see myself doing that from New York City. Then I heard about a computer bank in Washington, D.C., that was collecting the names of doctors and nurses interested in working with Cambodian refugees. I was in the process of writing my master's thesis, but I knew I had to go. I filled out all the necessary forms and waited. A couple of weeks passed, and I got a call from the American Refugee Committee (ARC) in Minneapolis. I was asked if I could leave two weeks later, in January 1980. Of course I could! I finished my thesis, got my shots, had my kids taken care of, and gave my beloved dachshund to my parents. Nothing stood in my way now.

Khao-I-Dang was the biggest refugee camp on the Thai-Cambodian border. (It's the camp in the movie *The Killing Fields* that Dith Pran sees when he escapes from Cambodia.) Some 140,000 people were living there in an endless prairie of thatch-roofed, bamboo huts on stilts. I was terrified the first time I saw it. I had never worked as a nurse practitioner. I did not know how I would react to seeing people without arms and legs. Paradoxically, I knew this was the right place for me, although I wasn't sure if I was up to the job.

Different countries and nongovernmental organizations were responsible for specific medical tasks. The American Refugee Committee ran the acute adult ward of 125 "beds," slung cots with reed mats for mattresses. Cornell–New York Hospital ran the emergency room. The Germans and Japanese performed surgery. Medicins sans Frontieres, the famous French organization, ran the maternity wing. Pediatrics had a smattering of everyone, including the English, the Dutch, and American missionaries. The

Italians had set up a mobile hospital to serve the Thai people outside the camp. The whole deal was very *M*A*S*H*-like, with sixteen-hour days, scenes of life-and-death drama, and scores of wild doctors and nurses from around the world.

All the Americans, it seemed to me, had come to Khao-I-Dang to escape their past. A lot of the nurses in my group were getting divorced or leaving sour relationships. Several were housewives from Minnesota who had never been outside the United States. Some scenes you would not believe. Women shared diaphragms with each other. An American nurse and an Italian doctor, lying naked in a sleeping bag, asked me to translate their lovemaking. (I speak fluent Italian.) One of the Americans was a nurse from the Midwest whose sweet husband and little daughter had seen her off at the airport. She got pregnant and miscarried. Working with displaced people as we did, sixteen hours a day, eighteen days straight without a break, threw your emotions into high gear. People went wild. When they finally came back to the United States, some of them changed jobs or left their families.

As for me, I faced a particularly thorny problem: Nobody except the Americans understood what a nurse practitioner did. I had been trained to handle a patient load and make diagnoses, but in Khao-I-Dang, I ended up doing bedside nursing. I had found that boring at St. Bartholomew's; in Thailand it was boring and overwhelming. Nearly everyone in the ARC pavilion suffered from dehydration and was on IVs. By morning the IVs had run dry, and the nurses had to start them all over again. Even more problematic, the Cambodians used to take apart the IV tubing and fashion it into handicrafts. Tending to 125 IV poles a night was utterly laborious, and because I had come to Thailand to work as a public health nurse, I was disgruntled about doing it.

How had I ended up doing bedside nursing? Marla, Cindy, and Linda, three American nurses who had served in Vietnam, had gotten me assigned to it. When the Vietnam War ended, these nurses had returned to the United States only to find themselves at odds with American culture. They could not adjust to it and returned to Southeast Asia. The three of them were top-notch clinicians, trained to work under adverse conditions. Everyone, including the camp inmates, used to stand back and watch in awe as Marla, Cindy, and Linda approached a helicopter load of maimed Cambodians, unstrapped some of them from the landing gear, and triaged the patients to the various medical pavilions. They were fast and independent, and they felt they ran the joint. When I, a mere American nurse, came along and expected to make rounds like a doctor, they were fit to be tied.

To keep me from making rounds, these three Vietnam vets arranged for me to work the night shift. Along with another nurse, I would run through a ward of 125 hospitalized people, dispensing medicine and supervising the young Cambodian orphans who helped bathe the patients, serve food, and pass out medications. Beyond the border, in Cambodia, we could hear the Khmer Rouge and Vietnamese shelling the outlying hamlets. And all the while, we had to keep the IVs going. Apart from the fact that the Cambodians would dismantle them, you also had to navigate around the five or six family members *per bed* who would stay with the patient.

I protested to Susan Walker, our ARC administrator. But she was stationed in Bangkok and was too far away to be of any help. I was so bored that I used to wander over to the surgery pavilion, where the Germans and Japanese performed amputations. I would also accompany Russell, a young ophthalmology student, who had come over with the American Refugee Committee to fit people with eyeglasses. According to the Khmer Rouge, glasses were a sign of intellectualism, a crime worthy of death, so people had thrown them away. Russell had set up his eye clinic in Khao-I-

Dang's psychiatric tent, a pavilion run by local medicine men. It was a very mysterious place. The medicine men prayed and dispensed herbal tea. I never could put my finger on what they were doing. In any case, I never saw anybody get well.

One night, after we had gotten everybody fed and medicated, we took our cots outside. We lay down under the stars and listened to the artillery in Cambodia. I thought I might take a peek into the French pavilion, which housed the maternity ward. For a place where women normally cried out in pain, the maternity ward was awfully quiet. When I went into the ward, I figured out why. The place was awash in marijuana smoke. In the delivery pavilion were six birthing areas, and every time a woman had a contraction, one of the Cambodian orphans would dart out with a joint and put it into her mouth. The women would take a big drag and relax. The babies were born slightly doped up, so they didn't cry either. This is how the Cambodians endured childbirth, and the French just loved it.

The French doctors were a riot. They were all Jean Pierre or Jean Paul, gods who swaggered around with their chest hair popping out of their scrubs. An arrogant crew, always on stage. We Americans disdained them, and they disdained us.

The contrast between the different medical groups was comic. Over in the Cornell unit, which was the emergency pavilion, you would see the hungover Americans sitting in a row, waiting for an early morning dose of oxygen to get rid of their headaches. The Italians had wine and parmesan cheese flown in from Rome to Bangkok every week, and if they liked you, they would invite you in for a heaping plate of spaghetti. Strangest of all were the Cambodian wet nurses. They would sit on these platforms *all day* and do nothing but suckle orphan babies. I couldn't believe it! They were like human cows. Yet they gave life to children who didn't do well on formula and otherwise might have died.

*   *   *

The Thais were angry that the world was showering the Cambodian refugees with pity and medical care. They allowed the Cambodians to settle into Khao-I-Dang, but they didn't exactly welcome them with open arms. Our medical unit traveled an hour and a half every morning from our lodgings in Aranyaprathet down a military road to the camp, and at the final checkpoint the Thai military would search us and our vans for contraband. They didn't want us to bring the Cambodians so much as a T-shirt. The government complained that Thailand too was a country with health-care deficiencies, and the Thais wanted the attention that the international community was lavishing on the Cambodians.

Here was my big chance. The Thai government authorized ARC to set up a Thai village project in which an ARC medical practitioner, a Thai nurse, and a driver/interpreter would go out to the villages and give medical care to the population. Nobody at ARC was free to organize this except me. After six weeks under the thumb of the three Vietnam vets, I was free to practice my diagnostic skills, as I had done in Egypt. The Thai village program was mine. I would get out of the camp three days a week and help set up mobile clinics in the surrounding Thai villages. These were places that had never seen Western medicine. People had never even been to a dentist.

All at once, I had the best job in Thailand! I got to see life in the villages and countryside. I could eat the fabulous Thai food. And I no longer had to do night duty.

The Thai military would send our unit into, say, five villages a day. Three times a week, I would meet with the head man in each village and ask permission to set up my mobile clinic, actually a little wagon. Before the head man let me set up, he would invite me to chew betel nut with him and his family.

Betel nut is a small walnutlike nut with narcotic properties. The head man would mix it with tobacco, herbal leaves, and some kind of red paste. We would have to put this chaw inside our mouths and chew it. I never could stand doing drugs. I didn't even like the high feeling I got from being on a Ferris wheel. But if I was to infiltrate the countryside, I had no choice. I had to participate in this betel nut ceremony.

The three of us in the Thai village program would sit down with the head man and his wives and chew. Inevitably, the stuff gave me a buzz. Once the buzz vanished, I started salivating. My interpreter, Shane, who had permed his hair to look like Donna Summer's, said, "Ms. Webb has never done this before." Everybody giggled in this hee-hee-hee way. I must have had fifty people watching me each time. My mouth filled up with red spit, and, like everyone else, I had to expectorate it. You're supposed to aim and spit between the planks of the teak houses, but my wad went every which way. Everyone knew I was a mess. They all expressed such good cheer, though, that I was allowed to set up my little clinic.

I remember a six-year-old Thai boy who came to one of my field clinics with his grandfather. He arrived dressed in his blue-and-white school uniform and complained of pain in his lower abdomen. He had not urinated in two days. I examined him. The foreskin of his penis had fused shut. I tried to open it but discovered that without surgical intervention, he would die of uremia, a condition resulting from the retention in the blood of constituents normally excreted in the urine.

As a gesture of goodwill toward the Thai government, the Italian government had set up a mobile hospital on the Thai-Cambodian border. Because I speak Italian, I had established a good relationship with the Italians, and they let me bring them some of my "hardship cases." I took this little boy to them.

The entire medical and nursing staff was getting ready to go into Aranyaprathet that night for a big dance. The atmosphere in the refugee camp was simultaneously manic and sad, and the doctors and nurses dealt with the horrors they witnessed by going back to Aranyaprathet and dancing and drinking Thai beer until the wee hours of the morning. I cannot tell you how many times I heard Donna Summer sing "She Works Hard for the Money." Her voice accompanied us from our residential quarters to the refugee camp, down military roads, and past rice fields. That song provided the soundtrack for villagers on water buffaloes, for men washing their cars in the paddies, for the doctors and nurses of every nationality. Donna Summer was our escape.

When I brought this little boy in, nobody was in any mood to tend to him. One of the surgeons agreed to do the surgery necessary to open up the foreskin. I saw him take a scalpel out. I was alarmed. I said, "Where is the anesthesia?"

The doctor said, "Don't worry. This won't bother him."

I will spare you the horror of this story. The surgeon was in such a hurry to get to the dance in Aranyaprathet that he mutilated the boy. The child screamed, and the grandfather wept. It was terrible because both of them had been so trusting. The child survived, but after this incident, I had no respect for that doctor. I never took another patient to him.

Four days a week I continued to work in Khao-I-Dang. Only now I joined the nurse practitioners from other American units on an asthma project. Asthma was rampant among the Cambodians, including our IV patients, women in Maternity, and children in Pediatrics. We finally traced the problem to smoke inhalation, a by-product of their food preparation. During the monsoon season, which, for us, meant walking waist-high in snake-infested waters, a haze of smoke hung over the camp. Moreover, the Cambodians may have been allergic to the smoked fish sent in by Catholic Charities and the World Food Program. With the backing of the International Rescue Committee, we set up a program to treat asthmatics on an out-patient basis. We gave them prednisone, steroids, and aminophylline, and in a few hours they were back in their own huts.

This is where my adversarial relationship with the three Vietnam vets came to a head. They were livid. How could I, a nurse with limited clinical experience, leave the camp three days a week, use an interpreter, *and* work on an outpatient public health project? They did anything within their power to sabotage me. They complained to the doctors. They stole away my interpreter. I would reclaim my interpreter, and the Vietnam nurses would take him back. It was constant warfare.

Our battles ended when Marla, the most bitter of the three, got dengue fever. It is a hemorrhagic fever that makes you bleed from the nose and mouth. Like malaria, it's carried by mosquitoes. We all took malaria prophylaxis and garlic pills so we wouldn't be a good host for the mosquitoes, and none of us got malaria. But there was no prophylaxis against dengue fever. You just had to hope you didn't get it.

When Marla was sick, I took care of her. It wasn't long before I felt compassion for her personal agony. She still had nightmares about Vietnam and tortured herself about the eighteen-year-old boys she had not been able to save. She had acquired a wisdom and understanding of the world that prevented her from tolerating everyday life in the United States.

Another of Marla's frustrations involved a failed attempt to adopt two little Cambodian orphan boys she had grown to love. They had nobody else left in the world, and they looked upon

Marla as a mother. But because of the adoption fiascoes in Vietnam, where Vietnamese mothers would thrust their infant children into the arms of departing Americans, and then try to reclaim the children once the mothers themselves made it to the United States, the orphanage administrators would not permit the adoption of Cambodian children by anyone but a Cambodian national.

Once you have nursed a human being back to health and seen her sorrow, it is hard to sustain an adversarial relationship with her. And vice versa. Marla and the other two nurses explained why they had resented me. They said that they had been out of the American circuit for so long that they had never heard of a nurse practitioner. They asked me to stay on in Khao-I-Dang for another month. I was burned out and ready to leave, but, for the sake of this new bond, I stayed.

Back home in the United States, after a tourist trip through Burma, I discovered that my experience in Thailand had bound me to the Cambodian refugees, the Thai villagers, and my colleagues. Like the American nurses who had served in Vietnam, I now understood what they were talking about: You had to see war to believe it.

Lucinda Webb is an adult nurse practitioner with the Women's Health Program at the Mount Sinai Medical Center in New York City and has done cancer screening examinations at the Strang Cancer Prevention Center in New York since 1985.

11

A Nurse-Midwife's Labor of Love

JANE ARNOLD

In the 1950s, a lot of people thought nursing was a menial vocation. The nurse—always a woman—emptied bedpans and took orders from the doctor. But I have always liked the maintenance aspect of nursing. Washing the patient, making the bed, and giving food are the cornerstones of promoting and maintaining good health. When you do these things for sick people, you are performing a life-sustaining service.

I entered the Columbia-Presbyterian School of Nursing at the age of forty-five when I was the single parent of four children and their sole support. Despite my financial insecurity and society's negative view of nursing, I had made up my mind to become a nurse. Juggling school and family life was hard, but as I have seen many times in my life, adversity is not an impediment if you want something desperately enough.

Take the example of one of my first patients, whom I'll call Carmen Ortega. She came to North Central Bronx Hospital to have her third child. Carmen had no legs. When she was an infant, her parents had left her "home alone" in her crib. The apartment caught fire. Carmen's legs were burned so badly they had to be amputated. Despite this disability, she had an incredible get-up-and-do-it attitude; if she didn't have legs, well, she would have to get through life without them. Carmen found a man who adored her, and although they had practically no money, she approached life with a joy of living.

I chose to work at North Central Bronx Hospital for two reasons. First, I wanted to work with midwives, and at the time NCB was the only midwifery-run service in the United States that I knew of. The midwives there did all the prenatal care in the hospital clinic. They triaged patients, delivered babies, worked on the postpartum unit, and consulted with the attending physician. Second, I wanted to work with poor, inner-city patients like Carmen Ortega, who come to city-run hospitals for their medical care. As a nurse, I feel a deep commitment to work with these patients. Wealthier women have a lot of options. Generally, they have good insurance coverage and can have their children in a hospital, at home, or in a birth center. The people who come to a city hospital, however, have fewer options. The city hospital is often their only source of medical care. It gives me a great deal of satisfaction to serve in a place where I am truly needed.

Working in places like NCB tends to destroy one's stereotypical attitudes about the poor. I know now that poverty does not imply a lack of family values. It does not imply a diminished work ethic. Being poor simply means you have less money than other people, and that's all it means. Most of my patients are rich in family togetherness, in love, in kindness, and in charity. They may be on Medicaid, they may live in subsidized housing projects, but as far as family feeling goes, they often have more than the people who live in the wealthy suburbs.

*   *   *

Before I came to NCB, I had done some home births, but working
on the midwifery unit terrified me so much I could hardly breathe.
For the first six months, people teased me about being "stiff" and
"too serious." The fact is, I was thoroughly intimidated by the
huge responsibility I faced. A university program cannot possibly
prepare you to do things like insert Foley catheters, so I ended up
having to learn by doing the procedure myself over and over again.
I remember that when I first came to NCB, I made the mistake
of eagerly telling my fellow nurses, "I just graduated from the
baccalaureate program at Columbia!" They looked at me, as if to
say, "So what?" They were right. My education had only begun.

North Central Bronx Hospital had its good-ole-gal network,
and I had to break into it. To test me, the nurses would give
me the hardest jobs. I was responsible for monitoring the
patients with gestational diabetes and hypertension and for
watching the women who were preterm and in danger of losing
their babies. I was assigned to a lot of cesarean sections, which
were tedious and time-consuming. Lunch hours and coffee
breaks were out of the question. If I got lucky, I might find
time to run down to the coffee shop. Most of the time, I ate
my lunch back on the unit.

The other nurses gave me every opportunity to fail. On the
night shift, I did get breaks and used this time to nap. I would ask
the nurses to wake me after fifteen minutes. One night no one
woke me. When I was late returning from my break, they said,
"What! You slept for two hours!" I replied, "But I asked you to
wake me up!"

I took everything those nurses dished out to me because I
wanted to be a good nurse. If they gave me a recovery room with
fifteen patients, I made sure I attended to each patient. I was deter-

mined to win the respect and trust of my colleagues. I kept my mouth shut, worked hard, and gave good care. That strategy saw me through those first six months of hazing.

Not long ago, the *New York Times* ran an article that lambasted the medical and nursing care at North Central Bronx Hospital. As a nurse who worked there in the late 1980s, I can attest to the professionalism of the nurse-midwives, whom I viewed as role models. What happens is that services like NCB get caught in the vortex of social problems, and the individual nurses and doctors are left to try to sort them all out. Yet no one person, and no one institution, can minister to the complex problems that arise out of domestic violence, drug abuse, unemployment, and homelessness.

What disturbs me about articles like the one in the *Times* is the impression they give readers about people from inner-city communities. It is true that it is hard to give nursing care to drug-addicted women in labor and delivery. People on crack are hyperactive; they hang off the sides of the bed and move around the room. They try to manipulate you into giving them painkillers. It's virtually impossible to keep a fetal monitor on them, and in the last stages of labor, they thrash around. From the nurse's standpoint, it is a real test not to feel angry at crack-addicted women. But persuading a woman to give up crack, and to give up prostituting her body in order to buy crack, is way beyond the scope of my powers. Therefore, I try to focus on *this* labor, *this* delivery, *this* baby, and control my anger at the woman who has chosen to ruin her life— and the life of a little human being who had absolutely nothing to say about the circumstances of its birth. However, these women and infants are the exception to the rule.

Most of the poor women in the Bronx care for their bodies. They come in for prenatal care; they care about their children; they are not addicted to drugs. This is the profile of the typical woman I see in my present job at the Morris Heights Birthing Center in the southwest Bronx. That's true of the African-Americans, the Latinos, the Vietnamese, and the white women.

Bringing babies into this world is a calling. In spite of the hazing I had to endure, my three years at North Central Bronx Hospital allowed me the privilege of witnessing dozens of miracles a week. Birth is almost like a ballet, with a series of movements so perfect they seem rehearsed. More than anything else, I have learned to respect the body's integrity. Regardless of the mother's social or financial circumstances, when it is time to give birth her body performs instinctively. And her baby automatically knows how to be born.

At times, my first year at NCB was a trial, but I would not trade my tenure there for anything in the world.

Jane Arnold is a nurse-midwife at the Morris Heights Birthing Center in Bronx, New York.

12

Beating the Grim Reaper

 SUSAN SCHULMERICH

The emergency department on Saturday night often resembled a war zone. On a Friday payday, many of the local citizenry would go out, get oiled, and wind up in all sorts of mischief. In 1966, I was a twenty-year-old, brand-new graduate on the evening shift at Mount Vernon Hospital, and I saw some pretty grim things.

One of them was a fifteen-year-old girl who had gone out drinking in a bar. When she came into the emergency department (ED), she tried to tell me what was wrong. But she had her hand pressed so tight on her mouth that I couldn't understand her.

"Take your hand away from your mouth," I said.

When she did, I saw that she had no upper lip. She had been in a fight, and her opponent had bitten it off.

"Do you have the rest of this anyplace?" I asked.

She didn't. These were the days before much success with reimplantation, yet we always tried to save the body parts. She was admitted, and I thought to myself, "They are never going to put this girl's face back together again." I don't know what happened to her. When you work in the emergency department, you see the horror but seldom find out the outcome after a patient leaves.

The bars were really big in Mount Vernon. The town, divided north and south by train tracks, is in lower Westchester County, New York. People didn't do a lot of drugs, but there was a great deal of drinking going on, especially on the poor south side. One night a seventeen-year-old boy came in with a bloody face. He lost an eye because he had been gouged by an adversary who used a broken beer bottle.

You couldn't always blame liquor. One night the cops brought in a little five-year-old girl. She was already dead. A stranger had kidnapped her, raped her, and thrown her off the roof of a house. The cops also brought in her killer. After killing the little girl, he had shot himself. He was alive when they hauled him in to the ED. Part of me said, "You're a nurse. Help him." And part of me said, "I hate this man." He reached out his hand to me, and I couldn't take it.

The emergency department at Mount Vernon Hospital was fairly small. There was one room in which to treat patients and one stretcher to get them there. But staff members were often very busy. One night a doctor and I took care of fifty-two patients, most of them victims of some sort of violence.

I worked there five years, in the days before crack cocaine and guns were prevalent. We saw a lot of knife wounds, alcohol-related traumas, and some drug overdoses. After that night with the fifty-two patients, I started to feel like God. I loved my kingdom: the emergency department. Some people say the thrill of working in the emergency department comes from beating the Grim Reaper. You are always doing this duel with death, and when you win, you go home triumphant.

It didn't take me long to learn that when your number's up, it's up, and when it's not, it's not. It doesn't matter who's on duty or how hard you try to save the patient.

I was in the ED when a freight train slammed into a school bus packed with children. It was awful. We treated fifty-one children, their bodies bloodied and broken. I thought, "This is like being in Vietnam." Then the ambulance tech brought in another child, the fifty-second. The child's face was not bloody or bruised. He appeared to be asleep, his body covered by a blanket. "What do you have here?" I asked the tech.

"He's dead."

The tech didn't know how the child had died, and I felt compelled to find out. I grabbed one of the doctors, and together we examined the boy. As I turned him over, I saw that his arm and part of his back had been ripped off on impact. By the time the ambulance techs had reached him, he had bled to death.

Fifty-one children had survived, but this little boy was dead. Why him?

Nursing has made me a fatalist. I believe people's lives follow a predetermined destiny. How else do you explain that one forty-five-year-old man who feels a little discomfort in his chest ignores it, then drops dead on the street from a heart attack, while another forty-five-year-old man takes seriously the little discomfort he feels in his chest, comes into the hospital, and survives? Both men recognized their symptoms. Why didn't the first guy act? When faced with this conundrum, I feel it takes a higher being to figure out matters like birth and death.

One of the most difficult nights I had was one Christmas Eve back in my beginning days as a nurse. A state trooper brought in two sisters who had been driving home when a drunk driver on the wrong side of the road plowed into their car. Patty, a third sister, died instantly. The other two survived. The trooper notified the parents about the accident but did not give them any details.

When the parents arrived and saw the two girls, the mother turned to me and said, "Where's Patty?"

One of the girls started crying. I looked at the mother and asked, "What did the trooper tell you?"

The mother believed that all three daughters had come to the hospital alive. I said, "Let's go talk to the trooper."

Now, the trooper would not tell the parents that their eldest daughter was dead. The doctor could not bring himself to say it either. I looked at the trooper, at the doc, and at the parents. By following my eyes, the parents understood even before I said, "Patty didn't make it."

The father became unglued. The mother, who was, for the moment, the stronger of the two, said that two years before on Christmas Eve, another drunk driver had killed their son. Lightning had struck twice in the same place, so to speak.

Christmas was not quite the same for me that year.

People have often said to me that because my husband and I do not have children, we have no responsibilities in life and we can have as much excitement as we want. After a night in the emergency department, excitement is the last thing I want. I want to go home where it is safe. My husband, who is a cop, feels the same way. Working in life-or-death situations, you learn that each one of us is here for a finite amount of time. And you know that tomorrow, if you are lucky enough to wake up, you will do the very best you can with the whole day and hope that the next day you wake up again. You never leave your house mad, because you never know if you'll get a chance to take back your angry words.

You also realize that life is far too important to take too seriously. If you didn't laugh, you would lose your mind.

I recall one case in particular that had a humorous side to it. On a cold February night a policeman brought in a three-year-old girl to the ED. She had been out riding her bike and somehow had caught one of her fingers in the spokes of the wheel. The finger was gone. She came into the ED with towels and blankets wrapped around her hand. This makeshift arrangement must have been six inches high.

"What's the matter?" I asked.

"Her finger!" whispered the cop who had brought her in.

"What's the matter with her finger?"

"It's gone!"

"Which one's gone?"

"The little one!"

"They're all little. Which one?"

"The *little* one!"

I crooked my pinkie at him. "This one?"

He shook his head yes. "Where is it?"

He didn't know. I said, "Do you think you can go back and look for it?"

The cop handed me the little girl and raced out. A bit later he came back, white as a ghost, with a quart-sized plastic bag *packed* with snow. On top of the snow as the little finger. The cop looked me in the eye, handed me the finger, and wham! He hit the deck! Here was this big bruiser cop, and a tiny little finger was enough to send him over the edge.

We beat the Grim Reaper that night, but we did not save the finger.

Susan Schulmerich is executive director of the Montefiore Medical Center Home Health Agency in Bronx, New York. Her most recent book, coauthored with Timothy Riordan and Stephanie Davis, is Home Care Administration.

13

Sixth Sense: Learning to Trust Your Intuition

PATTY TENTLER

In my first year as a nurse in Cincinnati, I had a patient named Henry Oslo. He was an older gentleman with lung cancer, and as the cancer worsened, he would wander around the hospital aimlessly. Eventually, we nurses had to put Mr. Oslo in a geri chair, a special seat with a tray in front to keep him from getting up and walking out of the hospital. Despite our best efforts, he was determined to be mobile. He would slide himself out from under the tray and go on his merry way. We were forced to put him into a posey jacket, a vest that zips up in the back and has stays that tie to a bed or chair. I would put him in the geri seat with his posey jacket on and sit him out near the nurses' station where the staff could keep an eye on him. However, no posey had been constructed that could thwart Mr. Oslo. When visitors walked by, he would flag them down and say in a lucid voice, "Excuse me. The nurses are real busy. Would you mind taking me down to my room? It's in this other wing." Some sympathetic visitor would go wheeling Mr. Oslo off the floor. He was so adept at escaping us that we affectionately called him Houdini.

One of the hardest things to learn as a new nurse is what to take seriously. In the beginning, I didn't always know what subtle changes signaled an emergency. In my thirty-six-bed postoperative unit, where I was an evening charge nurse, I had to be alert to a range of potential complications. When a patient first comes out of the operating room, bleeding or pain may occur. Vital signs need to be monitored. Anesthesia, for example, can increase or decrease blood pressure, so patients coming out of it are unpredictable. After two or three days, other complications can set in. A patient who has undergone bowel surgery may experience temporary paralysis of the bowel, which may result in excessive vomiting and more serious complications. By the fourth day postop, infection can set in and the patient may spike a fever.

Being vigilant, of course, was only part of my job. I also had to dispense medications, as I did one night when Mr. Oslo's call light went on in the nurses' station. Juliet, the secretary, spoke into Mr. Oslo's room intercom and asked what she could do for him. He said, "Get me out of this boat!" Juliet said, "Patty will be down in a couple minutes."

His light came on several more times before I could make my way down to his room at the end of the hall. I could hear his voice, demanding, "Get me out of this boat! I can't swim!"

At last I got to Mr. Oslo's room. I opened his door and saw the most amazing sight. A water main had burst, and water was gushing up around the sides of his bed. Mr. Oslo was sitting up, tied by his posey jacket to the side rails of the bed, and crying out, "I can't swim!" He was rocking back and forth as if he were in a boat. We moved him to another room and had the maintenance staff turn off the water.

That evening, Irene, Mr. Oslo's daughter, came to visit him. She sought me out and said, "I'm really concerned about Dad. He seems more confused than usual. He's talking about being in a boat!" I had to tell Irene that her father was not as confused as he appeared to be.

The episode with Mr. Oslo taught me not to take anything for granted: What may look like a clear case of dementia may turn out to be a case of eminent lucidity.

Many other situations demanded virtual clairvoyance on my part. One night I took care of Edna Baldwin, a coronary patient who seemed to be recovering beautifully. After I came back from dinner, something told me to go into her room before tending to other less stable patients. She was sitting up in bed and had just finished eating dinner when I walked in. She said something, and I happened to look up at the heart monitor. Suddenly, without warning, Mrs. Baldwin went straight-line. It was one of the strangest experiences in my career.

I began doing cardiopulmonary resuscitation (CPR) at once. As I pumped on her chest, she would wake up, but as soon as I let up to check her pulse, she would go straight-line again. For about ninety minutes various emergency medical teams tried to resuscitate her, but nothing helped and she died.

I have learned to pay attention to the sixth sense. A good physician will too. If I call a doctor and say, "I can't put my finger on the problem; the patient's vital signs have not changed, but I suspect trouble," the doctor will come. More often than not, a nurse's intuition turns out to be right.

A person's health can be such a fickle state of affairs. I have been on intimate terms with life and death for the past eighteen years as a nurse, so I do not take my health or my children's for granted.

Several years into my career, I moved to a transplant unit. I had a patient named Lewis Ryder who, until he was hospitalized, was a big, burly, healthy young man. One day he was playing softball, and the next he was so sick he couldn't walk. It turns out Lewis had a rare disorder that required a liver transplant. While awaiting his transplant, he took a turn for the worse. One of the L.P.N.s passed his room and heard him mumbling. She asked me to check him. I could not get a blood pressure reading on him, and his breathing was shallow and irregular. Lewis was dying. I feared he would not live to get his transplant.

I lifted the headboard off the bed so that I could get behind Lewis to perform CPR on him. I was eight months pregnant at the time and had to rest his head against my large abdomen. Some other staff arrived on the scene, and together we resuscitated him. We got him back! Incredibly, Lewis survived and recalls all of this clearly. Today when he sees me, he reminds me how I talked to him, and kept him calm, all while his head was resting on my big belly.

Soon after this crisis, Lewis got his new liver. Almost immediately, he developed a lethal form of anemia. With the help of a sibling-donor, he underwent a bone marrow transplant. It was touch-and-go for a long time. He lost sixty pounds and looked like a shadow of himself.

The last time I saw Lewis, his hair had grown back and he had regained his weight. *He looked better than he did before he got sick.*

When you witness the journey of a man from health to sickness and back to health, you know that something or someone else is driving his fate. You are merely the instrument of that journey, not the driver. In short, some people make it, and some don't. In other situations, I did all the "right things" for patients who seemed less sick than Lewis, and they died.

I'm not sure I could have survived my first couple of years as a nurse without the mentorship of my supervisor. I was twenty-one in 1977 when I graduated from my three-year diploma program, and Sonia Walsh was "just what the doctor ordered." If I felt overwhelmed, she would sit with me and help me figure out my priorities. She was supportive, good at problem solving, and, in a crunch, pitched in to help. Thanks to Sonia and my head nurse, I stayed in the profession for nearly eighteen years—even after my blind trust in hospitals and, sometimes, physicians, was shaken.

For example, I recall having had a patient named John Fouhey. He had just come back from surgery. From the start, his blood pressure was extremely unstable, despite medication. It soared into the mid-200 range. Despite numerous calls to his surgeon, Mr. Fouhey's blood pressure remained unresponsive, and eventually he suffered a severe stroke. He died in intensive care from complications relating to the stroke. When reviewing the night's events, the hospital administrators kept focusing on how many times I had charted my attempts to notify the surgeon. The implication was that I should not have been so explicit in my charting! Sonia and my head nurse supported me throughout the entire review.

Another patient, Richard Highstone, returned one evening to my floor after urinary tract surgery. While it was customary to have a moderate amount of bleeding after this surgery, Mr. Highstone nonetheless appeared to be bleeding excessively. I notified the surgery staff several times. They reassured me that the bleeding was normal this soon after surgery. It wasn't until Mr. Highstone's blood pressure dropped dramatically that I was able to get his doctor's attention.

Incidents like these were frustrating, but I did not let them sour me on nursing. Quite the opposite; I was always distinctly aware of how important it is for a nurse to assume the role of patient advocate.

Patty Tentler is a law student at Indiana University, Indianapolis.

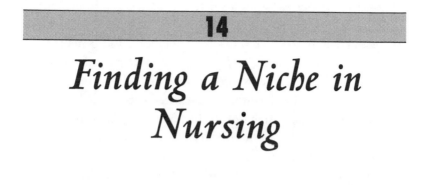

14

Finding a Niche in Nursing

DOROTHY STAGNO

When I was a little girl, my sister and brother were plagued with various illnesses. As a responsible female child, I watched the caretakers around me and felt comfortable assuming their role. In many ways, it was not that great a leap from my position as mother's helper inside my family to my desire to be a pediatric nurse. Yet during my six-week student rotation in the premature nursery at the Columbia-Presbyterian Medical Center, I discovered that I really was not cut out for working with severely ill children.

For example, I saw a baby whose mother had dipped her into hot water and burned her legs. I took care of infants with heart abnormalities or blurred sexual characteristics. One "preemie" was probably a thalidomide baby, with limbs like flippers. Her mother could not bring herself to visit, and her father would come in for an occasional five minutes. Another beautiful infant, born after a rubella epidemic, had only a brain stem and died after a few weeks. I was so sad about these children that I decided to work with adults.

Loss, I soon saw, was not a phenomenon limited to pediatrics. During a rotation with adults, two of my patients died in rapid succession. My head nurse told me how much I had benefited the patients and their families, and yet I could not shake the sense of alienation that began to envelop me. In 1966, when I first became a nurse, people did not consider that caretakers needed care too. Perhaps I, like other young nurses, had been influenced by reading wonderful "young adult" fiction like *Cherry Ames: Clinic Nurse,* in which the able Cherry Ames could teach diabetics how to take care of themselves, nurse her twin brother—a wounded air force pilot—back to health, and solve a mystery, all without shedding a tear. By the time I got to nursing school, I realized that I had absorbed a lot of useful information about medicine and nursing care from the Cherry Ames series, but I also had tried to adopt the rosy-cheeked fictional persona that never cried or got frustrated. When it came to facing real-life tragedies and frustrations, I, like many of my nursing colleagues, was left to fend for myself.

My attitude became fatalistic: "As long as you're in the hospital, I'll take care of you. When you're gone, you're out of my life." Sadly, this tactic had only short-term advantages. It took me many years to acknowledge the value of grief in the human life cycle.

My first job out of nursing school was at Presbyterian Hospital's Harkness Pavilion in the Washington Heights section of New York. It was a private medical-surgical floor with a few semi-private GYN patients. Like many new nurses, I worked the night shift, eight days on and, if I remember correctly, four days off. Working nights meant working alone. Although I sometimes talked to a private duty nurse if she wasn't with her patient, for all practical purposes, I had nobody to bounce feelings or ideas off of. I spent much of my time labeling blood tubes, recopying order sheets, and rewriting medicine tickets. Other duties might include sterilizing instruments, like glass IV bottles, forceps, and syringes.

In the beginning of my nursing career, patients used to stay in the hospital longer than they do now. Some nights it got very busy. Hospitals back then did not have coronary care and intensive care units; in order to monitor the sickest patients, the nurses put them right by the nurses' station. As the patients improved, they were moved farther down the floor.

Because of my isolation, I welcomed the chance to talk to patients. I still remember one Irish Catholic woman who was dying of cancer. Fiona Rogers (not her real name) did not want pain medication and got by on a little IV fluid. I couldn't do much for her at night except turn her over to prevent bedsores.

Mrs. Rogers would listen to the winds whip around the building from the Hudson River and say that they were banshees coming to get her. It was so dark outside, and the floor was quiet except for these howling winds. After having spent a day on the beach, and after having drunk several cups of coffee, I was rattled. When the night supervisor came to check on me, I told her about the banshees. She made me toast and butter. That calmed me down.

Another patient I remember from my first year was a Hasidic man on a med-surg floor. The nurses were told that, according to Hasidic tradition, a person has to be buried in the same position in which he or she died. In order to breathe, this poor man used to hang over the side of his bed rails. We were sure he would die in a contorted position. When he finally did die, he was half slumped back in the bed. The nurses straightened him a bit so that the family would believe that their loved one had died comfortably in bed. The family said how nice it was that the patient finally looked at peace.

Having witnessed so much pain and suffering early in my career, I acquired the self-protective habit of forgetting nearly all my patients' names. To this day, I can talk about those patients' diagnoses. I can tell you about their family situations. I can tell you how long they were in the hospital and the number of the room they were in. As for the humanizing aspect of individual names, I wiped them out of my memory. I wasn't being cold-blooded. I was only trying to survive.

In my third month at Presbyterian, I got salmonella poisoning from eating eggs in the hospital cafeteria. After I recuperated, I went back home to Pittsburgh. I got a job in Pittsburgh's Presbyterian Hospital as a staff nurse on a ward medical unit. While there were pros and cons to working here, like any place, I preferred it to Presbyterian in New York. For one, "Presby" in Pittsburgh permitted married and pregnant students to work and study, something that Presbyterian in New York had prohibited until about thirty years ago. To my mind, this liberty allowed for a happier, more natural environment. In addition, student nurses were allowed to mix IVs in their freshman year. At Presbyterian in New York, we had to wait until the last week of senior year.

I encountered my first medical ethical dilemma at Pittsburgh's Presbyterian. It centered on an older woman—whom I'll call Mrs. Brock—with monocystic leukemia, a rapidly progressing form of the disease that people can get in their sixties, seventies, or eighties. Mrs. Brock was taking Leukeran, a chemotherapeutic drug that was not working for her. She tried to persuade her physician— whom I'll call Dr. Scott Kaplan—to discontinue treatment. He promised to honor her wishes, but he went right on prescribing the Leukeran.

I talked to Dr. Kaplan about this. He said, "I understand what she's saying, but I'm just not ready for her to die." Mrs. Brock was a very likable lady, and she really meant something to Dr. Kaplan. It was hard for him to give her up without a fight. Oncology is a very tough field; the staff is always losing people. Dr. Kaplan wanted to keep some very special patients alive at all costs, even if they did not want to suffer anymore.

When Mrs. Brock caught on that we were still giving her the Leukeran, she refused to keep taking it. Dr. Kaplan seemed genuinely saddened by her death.

Sometimes we found joy in the most surprising circumstances. Miss Cherry, for example, had crippling arthritis. She couldn't sit up or lie down without excruciating pain. At 101, she was not a good candidate for anesthesia or surgery. The family, however, supported Miss Cherry's decision to receive an Austin-Moore hip prosthesis. I think they felt that whatever happened, it was worth making an attempt to end Miss Cherry's pain.

Amazingly, the procedure worked, and Miss Cherry's hip stopped hurting. With physical therapy, she got up one day and walked from her hospital bed to the doorway of her room. We aren't talking miles, but even this short distance was thrilling. Miss Cherry took a seat in the doorway of her room while her daughter groomed her white hair, and Miss Cherry just beamed. She looked forward to going back to her nursing home because now she was able to get up and move about by herself.

The most stressful part of my first year concerned my promotion in Pittsburgh to head nurse. I got the job over a diploma-trained nurse who had more experience than I. Susan Reed (not her real name) knew the hospital system and I didn't, but I had the baccalaureate degree and she didn't. The entire time she remained on staff, she did whatever she could to sabotage me.

Life was easier once Susan left, but I still had to handle a position for which nobody had prepared me. The workload was often overwhelming. For example, the hospital had a lot of part-time nurses who could not work a full shift. I had to come in an hour early to pick up the pieces. When somebody from the night shift left early, I had to fill in there, too. The day-shift nurses sometimes came in late, and guess who had to pick up the slack? On top of everything else, I was also responsible for scheduling and taking care of my patients. As a new nurse, I did not have the maturity or experience to handle the stresses and strains that came along with my promotion. I suffered through this job for a little more than a year and then was asked to leave. I was so happy! I moved to an NIH research unit in the hospital, where I found a more natural niche for myself.

After my tenure as head nurse, I realized that a so-called upward move had not enhanced my life or career. Doing research, and eventually taking various staff and teaching positions, suited my goals and temperament much better. In the end, leaving the head nurse position was one loss that, professionally speaking, was a gain for me.

Dorothy Stagno works in the neuroscience-trauma-rehab unit of Fairfax Hospital, Falls Church, Virginia. She has a master's degree in nursing and in education, and is certified in rehab nursing.

15

A Prison Nurse's Captive Patients

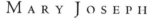 MARY JOSEPH

In Dominica, where I grew up, we always heard what a rich country America was. When I came to New York City twenty years ago, I had several jobs before finding my niche as a nurse with Riker's Island Health Services, and I witnessed first-hand how poverty shaped the destiny of so many New Yorkers. Riker's Island, a penitentiary on the Bronx side of the East River, houses 1,500 inmates and detainees from New York City's five boroughs. In the course of my tenure on the island, I have taken medical histories from more than a thousand of them.

From outside the prison, you get a unique geographical picture of the Bronx, Queens, and northeastern Manhattan: Riker's looks like a pretty seaside resort, with landscaped lawns, wild birds, and a view of Flushing Bay. On the inside, you get an equally unique portrait of the inner-city's poor, disadvantaged, and criminal classes, a stratum of people, mostly men, whose lives are shaped largely by drugs, sexually transmitted diseases, violence, and poverty.

Every day for the first six months of my job, I went home vowing to quit. Jail is not an easy place to work. The banging of iron gates and the officers' voices resound throughout the institution. The inmates are brought in dirty, wounded, and truculent. I would think, "There are better places to work." But something made me hold on. I thought, "What would happen if everyone felt as I do and just left? I must stay and try to make a difference in these people's lives."

At first, I felt thrown to the sharks. I would arrive at 7:30 in the morning, in time to begin dispensing 500 or more medications. At quitting time, I was still doing meds and requisitioning others for the next day. An L.P.N. named Linda helped me through the first few weeks of the jail routine, but mostly I had to figure the system out for myself. My only salvation was that no one assignment lasted longer than two weeks. At other times I would work in the receiving room or treatment room, which is comparable to a hospital emergency room. There I would handle a variety of medical emergencies: diabetes, hypoglycemia, hypertension, ulcers, drug withdrawal, and an occasional psychiatric episode. I also worked in admissions, taking a complete history, collecting specimens, and doing a workup of detainees before they were moved out to the cell blocks.

Some of the kids who come here for the first time are quite fearful. When I say kids, I mean *kids*, sixteen or seventeen year olds, in jail for jumping a subway turnstile or for selling a couple vials of crack. It's sobering to think that their three-day stay in jail costs $6,000, the same amount it costs to educate a New York City child for one year.

Two of these kids stand out in my mind. One had had the hell beaten out of him, probably with a "lock in a sock." That's when an inmate puts a combination lock into a sock or a shirt and beats a newcomer until he's black and blue and bleeding. The young boy I saw kept crying, "I want my mommy! I want my mommy!" I felt pretty bad for him. I couldn't give him his mommy, and I couldn't send him home.

The other boy had been given a six-month sentence. He was upset because his folks had not come to see him. I told him to write to his mother. He said he didn't have paper and pencil. I got him paper and pencil and told him to come back the next day so that I could tell him how Social Services could help him further.

The next day I asked the boy if he had written the letter. He hadn't. I asked him why not. The truth came out: He did not know how to write. I asked what he wanted to tell his mother. We sat down and I wrote the letter with him. Then I gave him paper and pencil and told him to copy my letter so that it would be in his own handwriting.

You don't know how many times I hear, "I'm never coming back again, Miss Joseph!" And the next week, bingo, they're right back again. The recidivism rate at Riker's is depressingly high.

I know that some people must go to jail. I once read a statistic that something like 7 percent of any country's population is criminal. But after working on the island for more than a decade, I believe that many people end up in jail because of societal problems, not because they are innately criminal. If you have no education, and no job, you may start stealing or prostituting yourself so you can eat. And if a society values designer sneakers and leather bomber jackets, a kid will try to get them at any cost in order to be somebody. If your parents are poor and you don't have a job, how else are you going to get those sneakers? When somebody in your neighborhood dangles a bag of crack or marijuana before your eyes and says, "Man, if you sell this, you can make a lot of money," you will see the drug business as your ticket up in the world.

This is a great country. But what's going to happen to it? We are raising kids who come into jail acting macho while they can't even spell their own names. Where are the future scientists, mathematicians, and other great minds going to come from? Certainly not from a bunch of crackheads, drug dealers, and jailbirds incapable of writing or speaking. As medical professionals and parents, we must begin to hold parents accountable for their children's actions if we are to raise kids that will carry this nation into the next century.

Mary Joseph is a nurse with the Riker's Island Health Services in New York City.

16

An ICU Nurse's Odyssey from London to Little Rock

S Y L V I A   M .   B A R C H U E

At the end of my three-year nursing program in London's Whittington Hospital, my job allocation officer asked me, "Where would you like to work?" Without a moment's hesitation, I said, "Ward 3." This was the gynecological floor, a unit with mostly healthy patients and a quick turnover. "I'm not surprised," said my AO. "You never missed one day of your GYN rotation."

The real reason I selected Gynecology was Sherry Brown. She was the unit's head nurse, and she made an excellent role model. At twenty-nine, Sherry was young and energetic. If we were short-staffed, Sherry would roll up her sleeves and get to work alongside her staff nurses. She also had an innate sense of fairness. Usually, if a patient was discharged, her nurse could eat the meal. In England, meals are served in specially heated carts, so the food stays warm. Sherry made sure that if one nurse got a free meal, all the nurses got free meals. Her philosophy was always, "One for all and all for one."

We handled the entire spectrum of gynecological conditions. One of the most commonly performed procedures was the prostaglandin termination. It is a biochemical form of abortion in which the doctor inserts a Foley catheter into the patient's vagina and up to the uterus and injects an abortion-inducing agent called Prostin E_2. This procedure may strike some people today as barbaric, but in the late 1970s, prostaglandin terminations were considered safer than vacuum suctions, which, depending on the stage of pregnancy, could rupture the patient's uterus. The truth is, doing abortions sometimes made me uneasy, and to this day, I don't know how I feel about the whole subject.

One patient from Greece really irritated me. She was a beautiful woman with a low threshold for pain. After nearly thirty-six hours of labor and endless complaining, she dispelled the fetus into a disposable bedpan. As I removed the pan from her, she asked, "What sex is it?"

I got angry. I wanted to say, "If you're so interested in the sex, why didn't you keep the baby?" As a professional, however, I could not divulge my personal feelings. Instead, I said in a clipped voice, "Does it really matter now?" The woman could tell from my voice and the expression on my face that I would brook no more of her questions.

Once aborted, fetuses went straight into the incinerator. The Irish Catholic nurses told us we were committing murder and refused to participate. Their decision placed a burden on the rest of the nursing staff. We came up with a solution: We would let the doctors administer the Prostin.

The doctors, however, were not game for staying up all night until their patients aborted. They began the Prostin during the day, stopped it at night, and started it up again in the morning.

This meant that more women were in labor for longer than twenty-four hours. We ended up using a lot of Demerol to ease their pain.

During my stay in Gynecology, one of my colleagues entered the floor as a patient. When I finished my shift, I went home to change and then came back to visit her. While visiting, I heard a knock on the partition. I peeked around the corner and saw one of the student nurses, whom I'll call Katy, beckoning to me.

Outside my colleague's room, I said, "What's going on?"

"You have to give Miss So-and-So Ergometrine," Katy said. Ergometrine makes the uterus contract after an abortion.

"I'm not on duty," I said and pointed to my street clothes. "Who is supposed to be working now?"

"Cecelia," Katy said.

"Then tell Cecelia to give the Ergometrine."

"Cecelia's in the bathroom."

"What's she doing there?"

"Vomiting!"

"Is she sick?"

"She saw the fetus move!" Katy whispered.

After I got over my initial shock, I gave the medication to the patient and then hunted down Katy. "What did you do with the bedpan?" I asked.

She had taken it to the disposal area. "Go back and see if it's still moving," I said.

It turned out that this fetus was dead. But several weeks later, we aborted a fetus that lived. The doctor on duty at the time took it to the neonatal unit. It survived, grew into a baby, and, as I learned later, was put up for adoption.

One of the saddest abortion cases at Whittington Hospital involved a young girl from India. She had fallen in love with a young man and wanted to marry him. As the parents of the would-be newlyweds studied their children's birth certificates, they discovered that bride and groom were actually half-siblings: They both had the same father. The girl had never known about her brother's existence until they began making wedding plans. By this time, she was pregnant with her brother's child. She had no choice but to abort.

The most bizarre case I saw was a seventeen-year-old girl with two vaginas. She was pregnant and required a curettage (a scraping process to remove tissue) in both of them.

Christmas Day was one of the most wonderful days at Whittington. The unit's three professors and their wives would join the nursing staff for Christmas dinner. The kitchen prepared turkey with all the fixings, and we each had a glass of wine with our meal. Christmas was the culmination of the staff's family feeling. In England, the hospital staff truly was a family. We did not bicker among ourselves. The nurses would not cut each other down either, as they do in the United States. And many nights while I was on duty, a doctor would bring me a cup of coffee. If I had to go to the bathroom, he would sit with my patient until I returned. I suspect that people outside the hospital world sensed our collegiality, because they treated us with respect. On a bus, for example, a person would give up his or her seat to a nurse.

One Christmas Day on ward 3, Sherry said, "Sylvia, there's a gift waiting for you in room one."

I thought it grand that I had two gifts, one under the tree and one in room one. What could be in room one? I opened the door and saw Sister Theresa in her bed, dead with a rose in her hands. Sister Theresa had come to ward 3 with uterine cancer. She was a petite French nun with whom I had struck up a friendship. In one of our conversations, she had said, "Sylvia, if you find a good man, shoot him!"

"What do you mean, 'shoot him'?" I said.

"Shoot him before he changes," Sister Theresa said. *"They all do."*

This was strange advice coming from a nun who had spent most of her life in a convent. But Sister Theresa was full of unpredictable wisdom. As I looked at her for the last time, I understood why Sherry had asked me to prepare the body for the morgue. She knew I had developed a close relationship with this patient, and I was the best candidate to shepherd Sister Theresa's body out of this world. Sherry had a dark sense of humor, but in her case, it only enhanced her humanity.

At Whittington, I used to mosey over to the intensive care unit whenever I had a chance. Although I learned a lot in Gynecology, particularly about ward management, I was drawn to the patients in the ICU. I loved trauma. It was exciting. I liked to work with patients who came in sick and, with exceptions, were better when they left. The best place in England to learn intensive care nursing was at Northwick Park Hospital, and when I was offered a job in its ICU, I was over the moon.

Northwick Park was a lovely world of its own. The hospital had a bank and shopping center, both accessible by a continuously moving, doorless contraption called a paternoster. The trains stopped on the hospital grounds, so getting to the theater district in London was easy. Northwick Park was designed with not only quality health care in mind but also staff satisfaction. The place was a dream.

Hollywood had just finished filming *The Omen* at Northwick Park several weeks before I arrived. As I entered these famous grounds, I thought, "Here I go again. I am the only black person in this group of lily-white people." But I had nothing to fear. I am not being obtuse when I say that I never experienced any hostility toward me because I am a native of St. Vincent in the West Indies. Indeed, my friends in nursing school called me a black-skinned, blue-eyed lady because I always got along with everybody. I believe that my professionalism and competence have shielded me from the feelings of insecurity that plague many other black people.

My ICU education at Northwick Park was extensive. The ICU encompassed pediatric, surgical, and medical units. On the same floor were a coronary care unit, the emergency room, and the operating room, and I spent about a month in each one. Having all the critical care areas next to each other allowed the staff to have a "Code T" system. Every day, one nurse in the ICU was responsible for carrying a beeper around. The minute the beeper went off, indicating a crisis situation, this nurse had to do whatever was necessary to help resuscitate the patient in distress. After the patient was stabilized, the nurse transported him or her back to the ICU.

Northwick Park stood right on the corner of an interstate highway, so the staff saw a lot of motor vehicle accidents. I saw injuries there that I have seen nowhere else in the world. The strangest one was a seventeen-year-old boy who was brought into the emergency room with his head sliced open on the horizontal. His mother had gotten him a motorbike for his birthday, and he had cracked it up on the highway. The oddest thing was that the boy was conscious and talking. We could do nothing to save him, though, and he gradually faded away. He left behind a guilt-stricken mother and a father who blamed her for the death of their only child.

Even less traumatized patients stood a chance of dying when

you least expected it. One doctor at Northwick Park was a fiend about vigilance. If he came into the ICU and found a nurse with her back to his patient, he would ream her out the rest of the day. His motto was, "Never turn your back on a critically ill patient."

To illustrate how quickly a patient's condition can change: One night I was working in the coronary care unit. A doctor and I were having a discussion when all of a sudden the emergency room called to say we had a new patient. It was my turn to handle admissions, so I got up to await his entry. The patient was about forty-five years old and complained of chest pains. Just as I wrapped the blood pressure cuff on his arm, he gasped. The man had gone into cardiac arrest before my very eyes. I thought, "Oh, my God! I have never seen this before!" Fortunately, the doctor was on hand to help me begin resuscitation. If we had not been on the spot, the man might have been a goner.

After one year at Northwick Park, I had had so much experience I practically was ready to help set up an intensive care unit from scratch. I met an American hospital recruiter, and he offered me a job at an Arkansas hospital doing just that. I had passed my national exam, so I had nothing holding me back from going anywhere in the world. Taking my first U.S. job proved to be one of the best nursing experiences of my life.

I always say that my stint at St. Vincent's Infirmary in Little Rock made me an ICU nurse. For one thing, the nurses there at the time were some of the best I have seen anywhere. For another, I had the privilege of working with Dr. Charles Nathan, a real stickler for patient care. He had the reputation for being a difficult man, but I found he let me enact the ICU regimens I had learned in London. The only problem I encountered here was from my fellow black nurses. One of these nurses, whom I'll call Dana, had been at the hospital for nine years but was frustrated that she had been passed over for promotions several times. She cited white racism as the reason for her slow progress. She seemed to resent the fact that even though I also was black, I was given responsibility for Dr. Nathan's open-heart patients soon after my orientation. Human nature being vulnerable to shabby displays of jealousy, Dana accused me of siding with the whites. I said, "That's crap. I want nothing more than to be a great critical care nurse, and I don't care what you guys think about that!"

The other black nurses told me I couldn't appreciate the horrors of American racism. They kept saying, "Sylvia, you weren't born in the South. You can't understand how we've been treated."

I felt that the black nurses did not push hard enough. In private conversations I would tell them as much. I said, "If you want to take care of the open-heart surgeries, you've got to be aggressive."

My work with Dr. Nathan was thrilling. Once an open-heart patient was assigned to me, the patient was mine from the moment he or she entered the ICU until I left for the day. I was responsible for monitoring the blood gases, determining the hematocrit, which is the ratio of the volume of red blood cells to a given volume of blood, and performing the lab work. If the patient's potassium level was low, for example, I had the authority to add more potassium to the IV fluids. And I had to know when the patient was ready for extubation, because it was also my job to remove breathing tubes from the trachea, or windpipe.

In the course of my American career, I have often wondered how the state of nursing came to be so chaotic. Did we nurses do it to ourselves? Although there are many nursing organizations, they cannot come together and agree on anything. Whose fault is that? We can't blame doctors, hospitals, or the health-care system for the inadequacies of our own profession.

Part of the problem may be that some nurses in this country

became nurses for financial reasons alone. They hold two, sometimes three jobs at a time. A mentally and physically exhausted nurse cannot possibly give good patient care.

You have to want to be a nurse to be a good nurse. These days a lot of nurses come out of nursing school with the desire to "coordinate care," "facilitate utilization," or "administer services." This is not what nursing is about. To be a nurse, you must get down to the nitty gritty. You have to do the dirty end of it first before you can become a glorified head nurse.

Today, as the head nurse in a Bronx surgical intensive care unit (SICU), I always advise my nurses to think of their patients as their mother or father. I hope they will give them the same care they would want for their own parents. Several years ago, I brought in four new R.N.s to work in the SICU despite a warning from colleagues that I was taking too great a gamble on inexperienced staff. The new nurses took my advice to heart and have become some of the best nurses I have ever known.

Sylvia M. Barchue is the head nurse in the SICU (Surgical Intensive Care Unit) at the Veterans Affairs Medical Center, Bronx, New York.

17

"You Stole My Tongue"

 V ALERIE K OLBERT

There but for the grace of God go I. That was often my attitude when I worked as a psychiatric nurse at Montefiore Medical Center in the Bronx. Before the era of biological psychiatry, our twenty-two-bed open unit functioned as a therapeutic community, and the nursing staff pretty much ran the show.

Between 1977 and 1982, I saw that the crises that brought our patients to us were not that different from the crises that emotionally stable people experience in their own lives. The main difference, we believed, was that our patients did not have the coping skills necessary for dealing with stressful situations. It was our unit's job to get our patients through the crisis and back into their community, and we hoped that they would better understand how to prevent another hospitalization.

Because we were a crisis intervention unit, we saw a wide variety of diagnoses, including schizophrenia, major depression, postpartum depression, anorexia nervosa, and borderline personality disorder. Depressed patients often had the most dramatic results.

With psychotherapy, medication, and/or electroconvulsive therapy (ECT), they would go from being actively suicidal—incapable of eating, bathing, or brushing their hair—to leaving the hospital thirty days later, ready to resume their lives.

Our unit's team spirit made working on "Klau 2" one of the best experiences in my life. The evening staff worked so well together that going to work felt like going to visit friends. Our unit was successful because we all valued effective communication with each other and with our patients. At our individual and group clinical supervision sessions and at our nightly team meetings, we formulated nursing care plans, discussed staff reactions, and worked hard to pull together as a team. Our supervisors treated us like adults. As a result, we usually solved our own problems. Our unit was one of the few at "Monty" in which the staff designed their own schedules. And if twelve nurses can work out scheduling without a fight, then treating a problematic patient is a piece of cake!

We saw a mixture of illnesses on Klau 2. Although they may have stemmed from various sources, sometimes all you had to do was look at a person's family to see why a person was "crazy." Adam Muller was a seventeen-year-old, newly diagnosed schizophrenic who spent time on our unit on several different occasions. When he was not hearing voices, he sometimes worked as a hot dog vendor at Yankee Stadium. Staff members occasionally ran into him at a ball game. Despite our protests, he offered us free hot dogs and moved us to better seats. It was his way of thanking us for caring.

During one of Adam's stays, Adam came with his parents to multiple family group therapy. Another nurse and I were leading the group that night while our supervisor watched from behind a one-way mirror. During this group, family members and patients discussed the patient's transition from the hospital back to the home. Adam's father was really down on Adam and blamed him for his illness. "What's this crap about hearing voices!" Mr. Muller boomed. "Why doesn't he cut it out and act normal like other kids! He could if he really wanted to!"

We understood that, underneath all his storming, Mr. Muller was really scared. But we still had to set limits with him. The family was acting crazier than the patient. Through it all, Adam was great. He understood that he had a chronic illness that he could control if he took medication and continued his therapy. He helped set limits with his father, but the tensions continued to escalate.

Without warning, Mr. Muller lifted his pant leg and pulled out a knife. He swore that he would fix Adam's voices one way or another. I was flabbergasted! Thank goodness my supervisor came into the room and helped us get the knife away from him.

At Montefiore, I lived in hospital housing, so I often ran into former patients in the neighborhood. One afternoon, I was returning from a shopping trip in Manhattan. There were no seats left on the subway, but the aisle was clear. Suddenly, I noticed a commotion at the other end of the subway car. In flies a disheveled young man, holding a hot dog roll with mustard, *sans* hot dog, rapidly repeating, "Geraldo Rivera, Eyewitness News," and shoving the roll into people's faces as if it were a microphone.

As is the custom in New York whenever a "crazy" comes through a subway car, everyone immediately buried their heads in their newspapers and hoped that this "weirdo" would not get violent.

I, on the other hand, recognized Harold Duckman, a former patient who apparently had discontinued his medication and was in the throes of a manic attack. I called to him as he galloped the length of the car. Looking a lot like Disney's Goofy, Harold exclaimed, "I know you! You were my nurse at Montefiore!"

Heads from one end of the subway car to the other looked up and then down again into the newspapers. I chastised Harold for frightening everyone with his inappropriate behavior, and I told him to stop. He did. He apologized profusely and stood next to me quietly while we discussed how to get his mania under control again. My fellow passengers gave me a round of applause.

Occasionally, we saw more than one patient from the same family. Sometimes their condition was hereditary; sometimes the family's pathological dynamics contributed to their illness. Basil Finn and his cousin Shirley, for example, were both diagnosed with borderline personality disorder. "Borderlines" deal with a problem by getting into an even bigger mess in order to deflect attention from the original problem. They are masters at "staff splitting," that is, trying to set members of the staff against each other. In this case, patient confidentiality was imperative: Basil and Shirley had relatives who worked at Montefiore.

One evening when I was in charge, I walked into the nurses' station and saw a strange guy reading Shirley's chart. I interrogated him because he was not wearing a hospital ID. He said he was a medical student assigned to Shirley's case. I paged the resident on call to check out his story. It turned out he was kosher. Now that I knew he had a right to read my patient's chart, I showed him around the unit and locked him in the quiet room to give him an idea of what seclusion was like. I told him he would have to listen to me and follow the rules if he wanted to get out. I guess he took me seriously because we ended up getting married. Working on Klau 2 really did change my life!

Ellen Brodman was a tiny seventy-seven-year-old Jewish widow with recurrent bouts of psychotic depression. She came in every so often for a trial of electroconvulsive therapy. After the treatment, she would go home as happy as a clam. One time, however, after three treatments, Mrs. Brodman refused to accept the rest of her ECT therapy. She became increasingly depressed and stopped speaking altogether. She had paranoid delusions and occasional violent episodes when she would turn my arms into her scratching post. One time she really tried my patience: She sprayed me with a mouthful of chocolate milk.

Mrs. Brodman's inability to care for herself, along with her violent behavior, made it necessary for us to draw up an elaborate nursing care plan. As her primary nurse, I took care of Mrs. Brodman. Nobody was pleased when I took a day off because then they had to deal with her. Eventually, even the psychiatric residents learned all they could from her, and I was appointed her primary therapist, a rare occurrence for a staff nurse. The average length of stay on our unit was about thirty days, but Mrs. Brodman stayed with us for six months.

Mrs. Brodman had no family. Her husband had been a jeweler and, from what we gathered, had left her well off financially. She did have a conservator for her estate who, we believed, was taking more than his fair share. Perhaps her paranoid delusions did have a basis in reality. One day Mrs. Brodman turned her suspicions on me. She came shuffling out of her room, her gait stiff from Parkinson's Disease, and gave me an evil look. In this shrill little voice she cried, "You stole my tongue!"

I was totally taken aback. Here was a woman who had not uttered a word in months, and now she was telling me, "You stole my tongue! I want my tongue back!" I understood the source of her suspicions, but all I could think was how surprised everyone would be when they reviewed my S.O.A.P. nursing note. The *S* stands for the patients' subjective description about themselves. For months, I had written nothing under Mrs. Brodman's *S*. That night, however, Mrs. Brodman's S.O.A.P. note started out with, "S—You stole my tongue!"

After a lot of political maneuvering, we had Mrs. Brodman transferred to Bronx Psychiatric Center, the state psychiatric hospital. A court hearing on her case was held on Klau 2 the same day I learned of my mother's death. It has always struck me as fitting somehow that these two relationships, both very different, taught me about dignity, compassion, and the value of caring, even when you cannot make everything better. Mrs. Brodman went to Bronx State, as we called it, with an elaborate five-page care plan. For a while, I was able to follow her progress through one of our attending physicians who also practiced at Bronx State. Ultimately, though, I lost track of her.

In nursing school at the University of Pennsylvania, I was idealistic about my role as a nurse. I imagined that I would spend time talking to the patients and teaching them how to cope with their families, jobs, and relationships. Frequently, however, reality intervened in the form of time constraints, endless documentation, and staffing crunches. Of course, nursing staffs should have such problems today! In my first year of nursing, our evening shift often staffed nine nurses to take care of the twenty-two patients. Imagine an almost 1:2 nurse-to-patient ratio nowadays in a health-care system strapped by budget cuts and downsizing.

In graduate school, I spent the better part of a year researching the different ways to diagnose schizophrenia. I wrote a paper comparing and contrasting the different diagnostic criteria. I floated the "outlandish" idea that perhaps nurses were also equipped to formulate diagnostic criteria, in part because they spend more time than anyone else with the patients. My professors loved my idea, but my stance was too "politically incorrect" to appear in a professional journal. The paper never got published. This has always struck me as paradoxical: Today, as more and more tests and surgical procedures are provided on an outpatient basis, about the only reason to admit someone to a hospital is for *nursing* care.

Valerie Kolbert is a volunteer mental health consultant at the Mothers' Center in Boca Raton, Florida.

18

The Twenty-fourth Evac: An Army Nurse's Vietnam Tour of Duty

BARBARA HESSELMAN KAUTZ

One of the biggest misconceptions people have about the Vietnam War is that nurses chose to go there. In my entire military nursing experience, I knew of only one nurse who went voluntarily. Her father was a career army officer, and she thought she knew what to expect. As for the rest of us, our reaction was just like any enlisted man's: "Huh? What? Me?"

The road to Vietnam began when I was eighteen years old. That's when I joined the army on a full-tuition college scholarship at the Walter Reed Army Institute of Nursing (WRAIN). In the summer between my freshman and sophomore years in WRAIN, I took a course in contemporary American history at the University of Pittsburgh, near my home. My history professor knew I had joined the army and challenged me to find out about Vietnam. I read about the Domino Theory and the other reasons for our involvement in Vietnam. I concluded that the United States was pursuing the only course of action it could.

At Walter Reed Army Hospital, where I did my clinical rotations as a student, I took care of a lot of young guys who were wounded in Vietnam. When I graduated from WRAIN in 1969, I had probably seen more guys with amputated extremities than the average civilian nurse sees in a lifetime. I have always thought it insulated me a little from the reality of being in Vietnam, and for that I am grateful.

By the time I graduated, took state boards, and went to the nurse's equivalent of basic training, I was beginning to have second thoughts about the war. Perhaps that was because of all those wounded soldiers I had taken care of. Perhaps it was the climate of the times. But I already knew that my first duty assignment would be at Letterman General Hospital in San Francisco and I thought I had upped my chances of being sent to Vietnam. A lot of returning army nurses came back to the United States through Letterman, which meant I might be sent in their place.

In basic training, the army gave us a good cop/bad cop presentation of the war. The Vietnam recruiter made the war out to be a giant Bob Hope Special. She placed a lot of emphasis on helping our boys and aiding the people of South Vietnam, valiantly caring for the wounded, military and civilian alike. The bad cop was a seasoned army nurse who told us we would be crazy to volunteer. Since I was going to Letterman, I decided to let the army make the decision for me.

The truth is, I was lonely at Letterman. My roommate lived off post with her boyfriend, and I did not care much for my head nurse. When I went home for New Year's, I told my parents how unhappy I was. They supported me in my decision to ask for an assignment closer to home or overseas. Before I could ask for a transfer, though, I got my orders for Vietnam.

When I got to work that day, the first person I saw was the assistant head nurse, Eileen Jankowski, who had spent eighteen months in Vietnam. Eileen told me I had orders. I asked, "Where?"

Eileen looked at me and sort of choked. She didn't have to say a word. I said, "Vietnam?" She nodded her head, and we both burst into tears!

I didn't bother putting on my scrubs. I went downstairs to get shots for tropical diseases and prepared to spend my one month's leave with my family. Going off to Vietnam was less than thrilling, but it sure as heck put an end to my unhappiness at Letterman.

The flight from Travis Air Force Base in California to Vietnam took about twenty hours. It was around ten o'clock at night when I sat in a Braniff jet, looking out the window and watching hundreds of nineteen-year-old PFCs stream out of buses onto my flight. I distinctly remember thinking, "These poor guys. *Going like lambs to the slaughter.*" I knew that some of them would never make it home alive.

As we entered Vietnamese air space, I needed to go to the bathroom. I got up out of my seat, but the flight attendant ordered me to sit down. I was not allowed to leave my seat until we were on the ground an hour later at Bien Huoa Air Force Base. Looking at the chicken wire in the windows of the arriving buses, I realized, probably for the first time, that Vietnam was not going to be a day at the beach. The sight of air force personnel with loaded guns confirmed my suspicion.

Later that day, we were taken to army medical headquarters on Long Binh Post. My assignment was the Twenty-fourth Evacuation Hospital just down the road, which specialized in neurosurgical wounds. I figured I would wind up on the neurosurgery ward because I had had a lot of neurosurgery experience at Walter Reed.

I was right. Neurosurgery consisted of two Quonset huts. One was a step-down unit with thirty beds. Most of the patients there were American, Thai, Korean, and Vietnamese soldiers with concussions. The other hut was an intensive care unit with about twenty beds. The injured there mostly had severe head wounds. We also had room for about six stryker frames, used to move guys with spinal cord injuries.

One of my first patients, whom I'll call Jimmy Matthews, was a young guy from Tennessee. Jimmy was a good example of what a wounded patient could look like. He had a depressed skull fracture, shrapnel wounds on his chest and face, and a broken arm and leg. We thought he might be blind. He was pretty much out of it most of the time. Whenever he did wake up, he would scream for his girlfriend, Debbie.

The neurosurgery unit employed a Vietnamese woman who acted as translator and nursing assistant. She was bent on anglicizing her name and would not respond unless you called her Debbie. Every time one of us called for Debbie, Jimmy would start screaming for his girlfriend. He lay in his bed, hollering, "Debbie! Debbie Lee Mae! Debbie, I love you!"

One of the medical corpsmen had a particularly rough time with Jimmy. Dressing changes were a battle royal, with Jimmy refusing to cooperate and the corpsman insisting that he had to. Out of desperation, the corpsman told Jimmy that if he didn't comply, he would sic Mighty Ralph on him.

Mighty Ralph was the bête noire of ward 5. If you had three patients who died in the space of an hour, that was Mighty Ralph's doing. If you spilled something that would take twenty minutes to clean up, that was Mighty Ralph's fault too. If your shift progressed without any mishaps, then Mighty Ralph was in a good mood. You did *not* want to cross Mighty Ralph.

I have always wondered what happened to Jimmy. I cannot find his name on the Vietnam Wall in Washington, D.C., so I assume that he did not die from his injuries.

Because I had seen ghastly body injuries as a student nurse, I did not undergo the same demoralization that other new nurses in Vietnam experienced. This was my job, and I knew how to do it.

I am not saying that Neurosurgery was an easy place to work. Permeating the air in the hut was a putrid stench. Nothing could mask it. The guys used to hose the floor down with water containing aromatic oil of cinnamon and peppermint, but it didn't help. I realize now that the smell probably came from rotting flesh.

We medical personnel did a lot of silly things, like organize spontaneous shaving cream battles or invent stories about Mighty Ralph. We did whatever we could to lessen the pain of working twelve hours a day six days a week, witnessing grotesque injuries, and watching nineteen-year-old boys die.

After six months, the nurses were entitled to change assignments. I figured I would tough it out in Neuro for the second half of my tour. But then one night near the end of that six-month mark, four patients died in rapid succession. I looked at Ted Harrison, the head nurse whom I viewed as my mentor, and said, "I don't think I can do this anymore."

Ted, an insightful, self-disciplined person, encouraged me to get out of the unit. By now, my attitude was, "What can they do to me? Send me to Vietnam?" Like many of my colleagues, I used to recite, "When I die, I'm going to heaven 'cause I spent my time in hell." A philosophy like this may get you through tough situations, but it puts you in danger of becoming callous to other people's problems. In dealing with life and death every day, we sometimes lost track of emotional subtleties. The grand-scale injuries we saw made a lot of people jaunty, even belligerent. Before Ted got to Neuro, the unit was notorious for its lack of military discipline. Enlisted personnel sometimes refused to carry out orders. Working with such horribly wounded young men traumatized the staff, most of whom were the same age as the wounded and dying. Ted, a thirty-five-year-old man with a career as a military nurse, understood this. I will always be grateful to him for showing me that to be an effective leader, you have to help each person solve his or her problems in a unique way.

I decided to switch to the emergency room. When the chief nurse found out where I wanted to go, she said, "Are you crazy? You're leaving ward 5 for the emergency room?" But Ted understood my intense needed to be needed. The chief nurse compromised by sending me to a step-down unit where we kept pre- and postoperative patients.

- By then I had become a trauma junkie. On the one hand, taking care of quadriplegics and young, head-injured men was demoralizing. On the other hand, nothing less than crisis satisfied me. That step-down unit gave me "the best of both worlds." Some patients needed nothing more than a smile or a "how 'ya doin?'" Others needed every bit of nursing skill I had.

This was the unit where I first encountered the concept of triage. We had a category called "expecteds," meaning "the soldiers who were expected to die." An "expected" took his place at the bottom of the pile, so to speak, and if he was still alive after we had finished working on the relatively less injured men, we would treat him. "Expecteds" had an abysmal chance of survival. These were the boys with their guts and brains hanging out. We would put them in a corner, give them some pain medication, and wait for death to come.

Incredibly, the staff also did some elective surgeries. One of them was on a young boy, the son of a high-ranking Cambodian officer. He had a spinal cord deformity that the doctors thought was amenable to surgery. Maybe it was, maybe it wasn't, but the boy didn't make it. We nurses were never comfortable doing elective surgery. Many of us felt that Vietnam was too risky a place to have surgery unless you absolutely had to.

Vietnam has never been a black-or-white issue for me. In the twenty-four years since I have been back home, I have had conflicted feelings about the war. In part, I believe that our country's involvement in Southeast Asia was one of the stupidest ventures we have ever undertaken. I also think I had no choice but to offer my nursing skills for this misguided cause. No matter what the politics of the Nixon administration were, the young men fighting in Vietnam needed me, and I am proud to be a Vietnam veteran.

I was at the Twenty-fourth Evac when Nixon invaded Cambodia. I had a peculiar set of emotions. I was upset by the increased number of American casualties, more than at any other time of my tour. Yet I also thought it possible that our incursion might end the war faster. I remember that one of my sisters wrote to me after she attended the big antiwar march in Washington, D.C. She wanted me to know that, in marching, she had made a statement about the wrongheadedness of the war. I wrote back to her, saying, "Don't do this! We need your support right now, not your protest."

I felt differently about her actions once I came back to the "world." My husband and I even gave money to George McGovern's presidential campaign in the hope that his election would end the war. Still, neither I nor my husband, a former helicopter pilot who flew wounded patients into the Twenty-fourth Evac, has ever been able to maintain a simple pro- or antiwar stance. I get frustrated with the revisionist historians, for example, who say we should never have dropped atom bombs on Hiroshima and

Nagasaki. It's true that the bombs killed hundreds of thousands of civilians, but if you have never lived through an endless war, you cannot fathom your leaders' desperation to put a stop to it.

My question then and now, however, remains the same: If it was obvious to the average nineteen-year-old grunt at Long Binh Post that the Vietnamese did not want us in their country, why wasn't it obvious to Richard Nixon and Robert McNamara in Washington?

Barbara Hesselman Kautz teaches maternal-child nursing at the University of New Hampshire School of Nursing.

19

Daughters of Miriam: One Nurse's Second Home

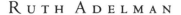

RUTH ADELMAN

Everything about my first job seemed ideal. In 1985, Columbia-Presbyterian Medical Center in Manhattan hired me to work on a medical-surgical floor. I was assigned the day shift, a relative rarity for a first-year nurse, and I could take the summer off to vacation in California with my two young sons. I looked forward to starting my job in September, when I could get some practical experience before studying for a master's degree in psychiatric nursing, my ultimate goal.

Within a week on the job, I knew I wasn't going to last. Instead of the two or three patients I took care of as a nursing student, I now had eight to ten severely sick people who required triple antibiotics, parenteral (non-oral) feedings, temperature readings, wound dressings, and clean catheters. One man had a horrendous internal blockage that made his belly swell. We nurses would have

to drain the fluid regularly and also minister to the many nosoco-
mial infections (infections acquired in the hospital). Another man,
an alcoholic at the end stage of his deterioration, needed total
physical care. His kidneys had failed; his belly was swollen; his
skin was yellow from jaundice. Yet another patient, who had had
surgery for cancer of the throat and neck, was thoroughly de-
formed and needed round-the-clock medical supervision for recur-
rences and infections. I was overwhelmed by the sheer volume of
work. Worse, I felt inadequate. My eight hours would pass, and I
hadn't completed my tasks. I felt terrible leaving my work undone
for the next shift.

On my shift was a diploma nurse who had graduated from the
Englewood Hospital School of Nursing in New Jersey. She was
quite a bit younger than I—I was forty—and had come to Columbia a few months earlier. Maddie Presser (not her real name)
had some of the most difficult patients on the floor, and yet she
finished all her work. I admired her. One day I asked Maddie
how she did it. She said that, despite appearances, she did not get
everything done, and she felt overwhelmed too. Perhaps because
of her youth, or because of her previous experience at Englewood,
she could handle the unrelenting stress of a hospital workload.

Meanwhile, I got on the bus every morning in tears. When I
got home, my son would ask how my day went, and I would burst
out crying. I kept thinking, "Another week or two, and things will
ease up." But the weeks passed, and I remained miserable. That's
when I figured, "Pay attention here!"

My head nurse tried to persuade me to stay. She showed me
my evaluation, which described my work as very good. I felt, however, that she had made an inaccurate assessment of my skills: I
knew I couldn't give my patients what they needed. Reluctantly, I
decided to resign.

✿   ✿   ✿

I took a couple of weeks off from my renewed job search to regroup. First, I called one of my professors at Columbia, a gerontologist whom I respected. She suggested that because I had liked being a hospice volunteer, I ought to investigate working in a nursing home.

By chance, I happened to see a news feature on TV about nursing home communities for the elderly. The reporter mentioned Daughters of Miriam in Clifton, New Jersey, a well-known, respected nursing home not far from my house. A week after the broadcast, I saw an ad in a newspaper for a part-time nurse in Daughters of Miriam's elderly day-care program. The pay was frightfully low, even for 1985, but I liked the idea of working part-time and going back to school for my master's degree. I was hired. It was just the job I needed.

Within a month, my schedule went from ten hours a week to fifteen. The staffing was in flux because the director of elderly day care got sick; the chief nurse took her place, and I became the staff nurse. Our small staff banded together in a tough time, and the administration supported us. I was also fortunate in having an excellent mentor in the new director. She was a patient advocate, always in close contact with the family and the physician.

At Daughters of Miriam, a nursing home with a medical day-care program, I discovered that I am a "talking" nurse more than a "physical" nurse. I loved doing checkups, taking vital signs, analyzing diets, and assessing medications. I liked consulting with the patients' doctors and families. The best part of my work, however, was being with the patients, most of them in their seventies, eighties, and even nineties. They loved to come in, sit down, and tell me about their lives. All of my patients had lost loved ones, whether to illness, accident, or old age. A lot were just lonely. And while you occasionally hear about the eighty-year-old who has taken up skydiving, most old people have to cope with the physical deterioration of their bodies.

The main reason I like geriatrics so much is that I get to combine the physical and psychiatric aspects of nursing care. The patients need a holistic approach at this stage in the life cycle, and they appreciate the nurse who takes that philosophy to heart. I feel I have always understood the needs of old people. When people ask me why I went into geriatric work, I say, "Because I loved my grandmother." Every day at Daughters of Miriam, thirty grandmas would search me out and love me! They wanted to tell me about their breakfast or their constipation or their toe. And whatever I could tell them about their condition made them happy. My job was to be there for them, and I was. Our affection for each other felt beautifully familiar to me.

Working with elderly patients has made me philosophical about the aging process. I have had the opportunity to observe how the elderly adapt to long-term illness and loss. Some patients "roll with the punches": When a spouse dies, they adjust. If they have to move in with a son, they adapt, even though they might prefer greater independence. Other patients get depressed. They complain that nothing will ever get better for them, and, not surprisingly, it doesn't. Some are reluctant to try anything new, and they often come to elderly day care at somebody else's urging.

I am of two minds about aging. On the one hand, I think you are who you are, no matter what your age. If you were an optimist as a young adult, you will remain an optimist into old age. If you always found a cloud in every silver lining, you won't suddenly, at age seventy-five, see the world through rose-colored glasses.

One time I had a session with three daughters who were trying to figure out how to handle their seventy-four-year-old mother.

Their father, who had always paid a lot of attention to Mom, was now a demented patient in a nursing home. Their mother had never lived alone, and the daughters doubted she would fare well in a retirement community. At the same time, though, Mom was so needy that she drove them crazy! I told the daughters that Dad's disability had not made Mom needier than usual: *She had always been this way.* The difference was that now Dad was in no position to give her the attention she required. I often remind families to think about what their parent was like *before* a health crisis, because chances are he or she has not really changed.

On the other hand, the physical and emotional deficits of old age do limit you. Either because I myself am fifty years old, or because I have been immersed in the daily welfare of a geriatric population, I am not quick to dismiss people who say that the "golden years" are not all they're cracked up to be. I try not to judge harshly because I'm not sure what kind of old person *I* will be.

At Daughters of Miriam, I lived and breathed my patients. In the car on the way to work, I would get a tensed-up feeling, thinking about a patient who had shown signs of heart disease, or about another who had dropped her dentures down the toilet once and might drop them again. At home I would talk about my patients all the time. Eventually, I began to relax. I tried to anticipate problems, like how I would change a colostomy bag or what I would do if a patient choked. And while I still preferred not to do physical nursing, I gained confidence that I could deal with any crisis that arose. The panic I used to feel in the beginning of the day began to disappear.

I stayed at Daughters of Miriam for two and a half years. By the time I left to complete my master's degree in psychiatric nursing, I was working twenty-five hours a week, a heavy part-time schedule for a graduate student with other clinical and family demands. Leaving was painful. For a long time, I actually mourned the loss of my wonderful "family." I know I had helped people by lending a sympathetic ear, holding a hand, and being a surrogate grand-daughter. But my patients had done as much, or more, for me.

Before I took this job, I felt like a failure; I had barely lasted two months on the med-surg floor at Columbia. I had been inse-cure and uncertain that I would ever find a nursing job that matched my interests and skills. But the patients and staff at Daughters of Miriam proved to me that I could be a good nurse. They even brought me out of myself. One day, our director pleaded with me to play the piano for the patients because the regular piano player had gotten sick. I have loved the piano for many years, but I had not played in public since I stumbled over a Mozart sonata at the age of nine.

After I played for the patients at Daughters of Miriam, I began collecting sheet music like "Bye Bye Blackbird" and "The Pagan Lovesong." And every once in a while, I, now a gero-psychiatric nurse, will tickle the ivories and make an eighty-year-old man re-member what it was like to hear Dorothy Lamour in a sarong sing, "Come to me when moonbeams light the eastern sky."

Ruth Adelman is a psychotherapist and the director of a geri-atric day-care center in Bergen County, New Jersey.

Bibliography

Boand, Nicole, R.N. *Just Beneath the Surface.* Long Branch, New Jersey: Vista Publishing, 1994.

Brady, Joan, R.N. *Fluff My Pillow, Bend My Straw: The Evolution and Undoing of a Nurse.* Long Branch, New Jersey: Vista Publishing, 1993.

Hughes, Lora Wood. *No Time for Tears.* Lincoln and London: University of Nebraska Press, 1946.

Laskey, Carolyn Travis, R.N. *Nurturing the Nurse on the Path to Success.* Long Branch, New Jersey: Vista Publishing, 1994.

Muff, Janet, editor. *Women's Issues in Nursing: Socialization, Sexism, and Stereotyping.* Prospect Heights, Illinois: Waveland Press, 1982.

Strangio, Linda, R.N. *To Be a Nurse.* Long Branch, New Jersey: Vista Publishing, 1995.

Suzanne, R.N., Carolyn S. Zagury, editor. *Ruptured Heart: A Caretaker's Journey.* Long Branch, New Jersey: Vista Publishing, 1995.

Van Devanter, Lynda with Morgan, Christopher. *Home Before Morning*. New York: Warner Books, 1983.

Professional Periodical

The American Journal of Nursing, 555 West 57th Street, New York, New York, 10019-2961.

Index

132 Index